DIABETES

The **Real Cause** and The **Right Cure**

Revised and Updated Second Edition

DIABETES

The **Real Cause** and
The **Right Cure**

8 STEPS to Reverse

Type 2 Diabetes in 8 WEEKS

Dr John on Health

JOHN M. POOTHULLIL, MD, FRCP

NEW INSIGHTS PRESS

Editorial Direction and Editing: Rick Benzel Creative Services
Cover and Book Design: Susan Shankin / Precocity Press
Text Illustrations: Tim Kummerow and Cristian Voicu

Published by New Insights Press, Los Angeles, CA

ISBN: 979-8-9860163-8-2 (Tradepaper)
ISBN: 979-8-9860163-9-9 (eBook)

Library of Congress Control Number: 2023921039

2 3 4 5 6 7 8 9
Printed in China

CONTENTS

PROLOGUE

IF YOU HAVE Type 2 diabetes, whether recently diagnosed or ongoing for years, this book will open your eyes to a new type of thinking about the real cause of your diabetes and the right cure that will reverse it. After reading this book, whatever you thought about diabetes will change. If you think that diabetes is your destiny because one or both of your parents had it, you will learn that what you have inherited is only a potential. If you think Type 2 diabetes cannot be "cured," this book will show you a completely different picture. The fact is, you can reverse high blood sugar and diabetes in as little as 8 weeks using the 8 steps described in this book.

There is a myth about Type 2 diabetes — that it is caused by "insulin resistance." Endocrinologists have promulgated this myth for decades, though it makes little biological sense and has not been scientifically proven. No gene for insulin resistance has ever been discovered, and no explanation has ever been supplied to explain why billions of cells in your body become resistant to just one of more than 50 hormones the body produces.

If you have been told that your diabetes is due to insulin resistance, ask yourself these questions. Why do only some people become resistant to insulin and not everyone? No explanation has ever been provided for that question. Why are only three types of cells — muscle, liver, and fat cells — said to become resistant to insulin? Why don't kidney, stomach, and brain cells become resistant too? If someone is resistant to insulin — which muscle cells need to absorb glucose to create their energy — why are diabetics able to use their muscles to walk, run, jump, and dance?

The answer here is, *because insulin resistance is not the real cause.* Where does the blood sugar go that your medications supposedly made disappear from your blood? Did it exit your body? No, much of the excess blood sugar is converted to fat that remains in your body. Lastly, if a Type 2 diabetic is resistant to insulin, how does giving oneself insulin injections help control your high blood sugar? This is illogical.

These are just some of the illogical and unexplained facts about the insulin resistance theory that you will learn about in reading this book.

So what causes high blood sugar and Type 2 diabetes? After 25 years of researching the medical literature, I have come to a more insightful conclusion that the real cause of Type 2 diabetes is staring us right in the face. It is our MODERN DIET, heavily filled with complex carbohydrates from grains that flood the bloodstream with glucose (sugar). Among so many cultures around the world, the modern diet is the only common denominator that can possibly explain the global increase in the incidence of high blood sugar and Type 2 diabetes. In this book, I will provide a scientific explanation for how our overconsumption of grains causes the body to develop high blood sugar and eventually Type 2 diabetes.

The benefit of recognizing that it is your diet at the root of Type 2 diabetes is enormous. It means that you can control and even reverse high blood sugar and diabetes by altering your diet to consume less grain-based and grain-flour foods. Let me put it this way: If you don't put glucose (complex carbohydrates) into your mouth, you won't need to worry about having high blood sugar. Doesn't this make logical sense to you?

Think of how liberating it will be to know that you can control your diabetes by paying greater attention to what you eat and consciously reducing your consumption of grain-based foods. Think of consciously reducing your consumption of grain-based foods. Think of the benefits you will enjoy by being able to stop taking medications or injecting insulin when you succeed in controlling your diabetes through your diet. Think of not having to get up from sleep with perspiration, palpitations, and panic due to a hypoglycemic episode. Think of not being afraid of experiencing the mental cloudiness associated with low blood sugar that happens in a Type 2 diabetic on medications. Think of the joy you will experience to be able to eat when you are hungry rather than on a schedule, or to be able to skip a meal if you want without having to worry about the serious consequences of hypoglycemia.

I hope you will take the insights and recommendations in this book to heart. Altering your diet is the single most important step you can take to avoid the serious and even life-shortening consequences of long-term Type 2 diabetes. If you believe that you are in "control" of your diabetes either because you can see your blood sugar numbers at any time with the use of gadgets or by being able to keep your blood sugar level in a desired range with medications, you are incorrect. The fact is, there is no other chronic medical condition, such as high blood pressure, high cholesterol, or asthma, where the patient is asked to keep checking a parameter multiple times daily and led to believe that this action alone can help control the disease.

My fundamental message in this book is: If you want to reverse your diabetes and avoid its serious and even life-threatening complications, the power is in your hands. The French philosopher Voltaire wrote, *"L'homme est libre au moment qu'il veut l'être."* (Man is free at the instant he wants to be.) This wisdom is applicable when it comes to being free of Type 2 diabetes, because it can be reversed when you choose to change your diet. If you are willing to try altering your diet for just 8 weeks, you will see your blood sugar level go down, you may lose a few pounds, and you will feel healthier and more active.

How I became interested in Type 2 diabetes

I am a retired medical doctor, having practiced for 35 years. I did not practice endocrinology — the medical specialty that deals with diabetes. But my interest in this topic prompted me to study diabetes from a different perspective and champion a different methodology for people to avoid or reverse it.

While I was in medical school, endocrinology professors told us to believe, as they did themselves, that Type 2 diabetes is a hormonal disease caused by "insulin resistance." I had no reason to dispute this. However, towards the end of my training, I came to know about one of my relatives who was diagnosed with Type 2 diabetes. She was injecting insulin to control her blood sugar. Her husband, a professor in a medical school, took charge of adjusting her insulin dosage to keep her blood sugar level within an acceptable range. Nevertheless, a few years later, she had to have one of her legs amputated owing to reduced blood supply to her leg — a well-known complication of Type 2 diabetes in many adults.

I then thought my relative's doctor would change her diabetes medication because taking insulin had not prevented her leg complication. To my surprise, her doctor continued the exact same treatment using insulin. Within a few more months, she had the other leg also amputated.

I started paying more attention to other people who were diagnosed with Type 2 diabetes. To my shock, I found many others who suffered severe consequences. For example, among my own friends were Dr. B., who was a practicing pediatrician when he was diagnosed with Type 2 diabetes; Mr. W., who was a researcher with a doctorate in organic chemistry; Mr. J., who was a successful businessman; Mrs. K., who was a nurse; and Mrs. R., who was a mother of five children.

Everyone mentioned above did what their endocrinologists told them to do. No endocrinologist told them why taking insulin made sense if their cells were resistant to insulin. No endocrinologist warned them that taking insulin would not prevent one or more of the many debilitating complications of Type 2 diabetes. Yet, the results were as follows: Dr. B. suffered a massive heart attack from blockage caused by fat, most likely produced by his liver from the glucose that was removed from the blood as a result of the insulin he injected into his body. Mr. W. developed cancer, because insulin stimulates the growth of cancer cells. Mr. J. developed vision damage and needed frequent visits to the eye doctor. Mrs. K. experienced the failure of both kidneys, needing permanent dialysis for survival. Mrs. R. developed Alzheimer's, a known complication of Type 2 diabetes.

I wondered how this could be. Despite taking medications or injecting insulin, I was shocked that these patients had still suffered the consequences of long-term diabetes. About 25 years ago, I began intently studying the medical literature on hunger, weight gain, obesity, and diabetes.

Through my research, I came to the surprising conclusion that this book teaches you — *the theory of "insulin resistance" is illogical and also remains scientifically unproved.* I know I am going against decades of medical tradition, but I am committed to asking questions and raising public awareness about the real cause and the right cure for Type 2 diabetes.

Diabetes is fast becoming an epidemic in the United States and in many Western countries. By 2050, it is predicted that one-third of all US adults will have Type 2 diabetes. The costs for treating so many millions of diabetes patients, currently $1 out of every $4 spent on healthcare in the US, will skyrocket. The insulin resistance theory, however, is what endocrinologists believe in; it is the rationale they use to keep prescribing medications including insulin injections to diabetic patients.

What is ironic, however, is that endocrinologists increasingly admit that diet and exercise are vital factors in controlling high blood sugar. This admission is a recent development, which I surmise is because it has become obvious to the medical profession that relying on oral medications and insulin injections alone does not effectively prevent the long-term consequences of Type 2 diabetes. It is truly short-sighted that endocrinologists still counsel their patients to rely mostly on oral medications or insulin injections which continue to promote the insulin resistance theory rather than accepting the fundamental fact that a low-carbohydrate diet is the most effective way to control and reverse Type 2 diabetes.

Sometimes scientific theories need to be updated

There are times when existing science turns out to be wrong, and the insulin resistance explanation for the cause of Type 2 diabetes is one of them. For more than 80 years, it has been accepted that high blood sugar is caused by insulin resistance, a condition in which certain cells in the body are no longer sensitive to the presence of insulin and therefore these cells stop allowing glucose to enter.

Using this theory, patients are led to believe that such insulin resistance cannot be reversed once it starts. This sets off a chain of actions, starting with taking oral medications, increasing their dosage, changing to stronger and stronger medications, and eventually giving oneself insulin injections, often multiple times daily. Or, patients may be given medications that cause the release of insulin from their own pancreas based on the prevailing blood sugar level.

However, you should be aware that the insulin resistance theory has never been proved as biological fact. The theory has never explained why the loss of insulin sensitivity in cells occurs, or by what biological mechanism the loss takes place. The theory cannot explain why younger and younger children develop insulin resistance, leading to high blood sugar and diabetes in pre-teens and teens as young as 12, 13, and 14. The theory cannot explain why thin people as well as those who are overweight develop diabetes. It fails to explain why some pregnant women can develop gestational diabetes within 8 weeks of pregnancy and then, within days after giving birth, their diabetes disappears. As you will learn in this book, there are too many inconsistencies and logical leaps of medical science for us to continue believing in insulin resistance.

After critically examining decades of the research, I have developed a new, more understandable explanation for the cause of high blood sugar and diabetes. It answers the above questions about younger and younger children developing diabetes, about thin and overweight people equally getting it, and about some pregnant women becoming subject to gestational diabetes. My explanation for the cause of high blood sugar and diabetes also sheds light on why diabetes is spreading throughout the world, as millions of people are now developing it. And most importantly, my explanation for the cause of high blood sugar and Type 2 diabetes provides the answer to how it can actually be reversed. In short, I will show you how your diabetes can be "cured" if you follow the 8 steps that are explained in this book.

Here is the key to what you need to understand. High blood sugar and diabetes are caused by the constant consumption of grains and grain-flour products more than what your body can utilize. Your body's natural process is to convert excess carbohydrate consumption, absorbed into the body as glucose from the intestine, into fatty acids to be stored as fat. But eventually, if you over-consume grains, you fill your body's fat cells. When they reach their capacity, your fat cells become unable to accommodate any further fatty acids for storage. This event leaves the fatty acids in the blood, triggering your muscle cells to switch from burning glucose to burning those fatty acids, which they easily do.

The result: You end up with excess glucose accumulating in your bloodstream, leading to the diagnosis of high blood sugar, and eventually Type 2 diabetes.

This explanation about the real cause of diabetes opens new avenues for how you can reverse it if you have already been diagnosed. It allows doctors to treat your diabetes earlier and better, without them resorting to prescribing medications taken by mouth or injected into the body. Medications do not, in fact, eliminate the dire consequences of diabetes. They may drive glucose out of the blood, but not out of the body (unless you are taking medications that block the reabsorption of glucose in the kidney tubules).

When glucose remains in your body, as it does when you have diabetes, it can lead to serious health complications including blindness, heart attack, stroke, kidney failure, amputation, and more. Also, it is far more dangerous to experience extreme low blood sugar induced by medications than slightly elevated blood sugar for short periods of time. In addition, medications that promote excretion of glucose through the urine increase the risk of ketoacidosis, urinary tract infections, and candida vulvovaginitis.

Just 8 STEPS to cure diabetes?

Curing diabetes means reducing a high blood sugar level to below the diabetic threshold (after a 12-hour fast, a range of 70.2 to 100 mg/dl is considered normal) and keeping it below that level on an ongoing basis to avoid its severe complications. Is it possible to do this in just 8 steps? The answer is yes.

This book will show you the critical 8 steps that will change your life in the most convenient way possible, helping you reverse your diabetes.* While you may believe that eliminating grains from your diet

---

* Reversing diabetes will not repair any damage the disease might have already caused, such as damage to your nerves (diabetic neuropathy), eye problems, kidney problems, or heart problems. Once the cells of the body are damaged owing to diabetes, the damage is usually irreversible. But this does not imply you should not reverse your ongoing diabetes. Lowering your high blood sugar may prevent further damage and other consequences.

will be difficult, if not impossible, these 8 steps will teach you how it can be done in a way that makes you feel motivated, proud, and increasingly healthy, rather than as if you are suffering or are being deprived of foods you love.

Just as you do not consult a package, a chart, or a book to determine how much to drink when you are thirsty, I do not prescribe what you can eat when you are hungry. These 8 steps are not a "diet" per se, but a revitalization of your lifestyle choices in favor of reconnecting with your "authentic" weight. I teach you how you can relearn to eat only when you are truly hungry, avoiding overeating and reimagining the value of good food in your life. Except for avoiding grains as much as possible, I will show how you can eat nearly every food, savoring its flavors and textures, and the delicious experience of enjoying every meal.

If, despite taking medications, your fasting blood sugar level has been going up, the recommendations in this book will help lower your high blood sugar. Changing your lifestyle habits to reduce your grain consumption as much as possible, based on the new theory in this book about the real cause of diabetes, will help you avoid the progression of your diabetes and its many complications. This will potentially save your life.

Just 8 WEEKS to cure diabetes?

Yes, by following the 8 steps in this book, most people can significantly lower their blood sugar within as few as 8 weeks or less.**

It does not take years to begin emptying your fat cells that have stored excess glucose (in the form of fatty acids) if you reduce your consumption of grains and grain-based products. As soon as the fatty acid level is normalized in your blood, your cells will revert to burning

---

** People with very high blood sugar level may take longer than 8 weeks. People with damaged pancreatic cells may have difficulty maintaining blood sugar level.

glucose, thus lowering your blood sugar, and very likely helping you lose weight as well. Working in unison with your doctor, you may be able to curtail taking an oral diabetes medication such as a pill, or if you are taking insulin injections, you will likely be able to lower the dosage little by little to zero.

Is there any proof that such a change in blood sugar can occur so quickly? The answer is, yes; one significant scientific experiment has shown that blood sugar can be reduced in as little as 8 weeks once there is a diet change that includes avoiding complex carbohydrates such as grains. You will read about that experiment in detail in Part I of the book.

I invite you to try out the 8 steps in this book for the period of 8 weeks. These steps work together as a complete program to lower your blood sugar, reconnect with your body and the right weight for you, relearn how to eat for health while enjoying your food, and avoid the destructive patterns of overeating, gaining weight, and creating an unhealthy lifestyle.

GRAINS
THE REAL CAUSE OF
TYPE 2 DIABETES

THE LINK BETWEEN GRAINS AND DIABETES

CHANCES ARE you already know that to control your diabetes, you should exercise and eat a "healthy diet" with more fresh vegetables and fewer carbohydrates. If you already have diabetes, you may also be taking a pill or injecting insulin to control it, but your doctor has probably given you this advice to exercise and eat a healthy diet.

This seems like common sense, right? If you eat a healthy diet, you won't put on any pounds. If you don't gain weight, you likely will be better able to control your diabetes since the two are highly correlated.

So why do you need this book?

One good answer is that, if you are like an increasing number of people in the world, you usually do not follow such advice. You continue to eat carbohydrates (you may not even be certain which foods contain those "bad" carbs). At parties, celebrations, holidays, and perhaps a few meals per week, you may also knowingly overeat, unable to control your attraction to food that looks and tastes so good. You promise yourself that you will make up for eating more today by eating less tomorrow . . . but you don't adhere to this promise. And as you get older, you may exercise less because you are busy with work, family, and social obligations. So you begin gaining weight; for many people,

3

this contributes to developing high blood sugar and diabetes. Getting inspired to learn how NOT to continue gaining weight and to reverse your diabetes is enough of a good reason to read this book.

But there is an even more important reason — the common-sense medical advice is largely wrong about why you need to avoid carbohydrates to reverse weight gain and diabetes. It is also wrong about giving you the impression that exercise can help you lose weight (it generally cannot) versus teaching you the real benefits of exercise for your health.

My goal is to explain to you the correct reasons why you want to eat healthier foods, avoid carbohydrates, and use exercise to condition your body but not for losing weight. Learning this information can make a real difference in successfully changing your lifestyle habits and feeling motivated to stick to healthier new ones.

In my experience, I find that when people know and understand the most logical explanation for why they gain weight, develop high blood sugar, and eventually have a full-blown case of diabetes, they are far more willing to abandon unscientific thinking and emotional rationalization than to keep living with the same bad habits.

Understanding this book can make a difference if you have been diagnosed with diabetes because you will see that you can take specific steps to reverse your high blood sugar. You may even be able to stop taking diabetic medications or lower the dosage of your insulin injections. If you are worried about your diabetes, and want to do something about it, you will find this book your valuable guide to a new life of health and vitality, without high blood sugar and diabetes-related complications.

What is Type 2 diabetes?

Just to be clear, let's define what is meant by diabetes in this book. First, there are two common forms of diabetes:

Type 1 diabetes — In this form of diabetes, the special cells in the pancreas that are responsible for producing insulin do not function adequately. Insulin is the hormone messenger that tells the body's cells to allow glucose from the bloodstream into them. The cells use glucose to produce the energy they need for their normal functions. In general, Type 1 diabetes occurs when people develop a non-functioning pancreas, most often starting in infancy or sometimes years after birth. Type 1 diabetes is a real disease.

Type 2 diabetes — In this form of diabetes, it is currently believed that either the pancreas does not produce enough insulin relative to the amount of glucose in the blood or that the insulin is ineffective, so the body's cells do not take in glucose. This leaves glucose in the bloodstream, thus high blood sugar.

The problem with high blood sugar is that excessive amounts of glucose can cause damage to various types of cells in the body, including nerve cells and cells in the blood vessels, heart, kidney, and eyes. These can lead to dangerous and even life-threatening conditions (see sidebar on next page on why you don't want to have diabetes). This book is about Type 2 diabetes and explains exactly why its cause has been misunderstood and needs to be updated. This is the information that will help you successfully change your lifestyle and eating habits to reverse your diabetes.

A simple logical question is the tipoff

Look at these facts:

- According to the International Diabetes Federation, 435 million people worldwide had Type 2 diabetes in 2023. This is expected to rise to 630 million people by 2030.

Why you don't want to have diabetes!

Most people never imagine they might develop diabetes, especially when you are only in your 20s or 30s. Even if diabetes is in your family — such as a parent, grandparent, aunt, or uncle — you may have believed that it could not happen to you. But the fact is, the incidence of diabetes is rising rapidly, at younger and younger ages. Today, teenagers, youth of the Millennial generation, and adults of all ages are being diagnosed with high blood sugar (pre-diabetes) and full-blown diabetes. We'll discuss the reasons for the sharp rise in diabetes shortly, but for now, just take in the repercussions of having diabetes.

Diabetes is a serious medical condition. Below are some of the health problems that uncontrolled Type 2 diabetes causes:

- *Dehydration.* The buildup of sugar in the blood causes an increase in urination, which can lead to dehydration and complications stemming from that.
- *Damage to body cells.* When blood glucose levels consistently stay high, glucose can get attached to proteins of cells such as nerve cells, interfering with their function.
- *Potential organ failure.* Uncontrolled glucose levels in the blood damage the small blood vessels in the eyes and kidneys, possibly leading to blindness or kidney failure.
- *Atherosclerosis.* Diabetes can lead to hardening of the arteries, which can cause heart attacks and stroke.
- *Diabetic coma.* A person with Type 2 diabetes who becomes severely dehydrated and is unable to drink enough fluids to make up for the fluid losses can go into a diabetic coma.

Decades ago, Type 2 diabetes was called "adult onset" because the typical age of onset was over 60 years. Today, people in their 30s or 40s get diabetes. Some children are even diagnosed as early as their teens. Once you get high blood sugar, it can persist throughout your lifetime unless you do something to reverse it. But you can cure your diabetes in a completely natural way if you follow the concepts and advice in this book.

- In the US, about 12% of the adult population has diabetes, and more than one-third of adults over 20 years of age have prediabetes, which can become full diabetes within five years. These statistics represent a huge increase since 1980.
- In the US, 1,560 children under the age of 19 years were diagnosed with Type 2 diabetes in 2021.
- The incidence of Type 2 diabetes has risen in nearly every nation of the world, including in many low and middle-income countries, such as India and China.

Consider this question: What connects these statistics? Why are more and more people throughout the world developing diabetes, given that it is not a contagious disease? Logic dictates that some factor must be driving the increase. Might it be that some people are evolving to be unable to process glucose? That seems illogical and unlikely, given that evolution does not happen in 40 or 50 years, and that not every human on earth is evolving to experience the same problem.

After more than 25 years of research, I am convinced that the cause of the rising incidence of diabetes is *the consumption of grains and grain-flour products*. There can be no doubt about this: the linkage is clear. As more and more nations have come to depend on grains as the leading staple of their diet, the incidence of Type 2 diabetes has correspondingly risen. This is evident in the US where the increasing incidence of weight gain and associated conditions such as Type 2 diabetes is easily documented.

Given the above, it's clear the culprit is the increase in the consumption of grains found in fast foods, packaged foods and snacks, and grain-flour bakery goods.[1] Similarly, it is evident in countries like India and China, where their growing middle-class populations consume more white rice than before and, in recent decades, more people are consuming fast foods and sweets.

Humans were not meant to eat so much grain!

The ancestors of modern humans *(homo sapiens)* appeared about 300,000 years ago and lived a "hunter-gatherer" lifestyle, surviving on meat, fruits, and vegetables. Consumption of wild grains started only after about 200,000 years of modern human existence and the domestication of rice and grains like wheat and rye dates back to only about 10,000 BCE. This means that humans survived without consuming significant amounts of grain and grain products for the vast majority of human life on earth.

Humans were always equipped to break down complex carbohydrates. But it's likely that early humans obtained complex carbohydrates and carbohydrate-associated nutrients from vegetables that required chewing, such as yam, cassava, potato, and taro. It was not until several millennia ago that carbohydrates from grains became a staple of the human diet.

In the Middle Ages, many cultures survived on porridge, rice, or potatoes, depending on which of these crops grew in their region. In the late 19th century, industrialized roller mills were invented, making it easier and cheaper to refine grains into flour for bread and other products made with starches and flours. Because of this, grains eventually became the major source of carbohydrates in human diets.

But in the last century, as never before, modern agricultural practices have altered grain agriculture and the production of grain products, fueling a tremendous increase in the primary role of grains in our diets.

Today, agricultural science has allowed us to cultivate hybridized, drought-resistant grain crops using irrigation, fertilizer, and machinery to produce an abundance of carbohydrates to feed humanity. The top three crops produced in the world are corn, rice, and wheat. During the 2021/22 season, 1.2 billion metric tons of corn, 787 million metric tons of rice, and 778 million metric tons of wheat were produced. This production is supposedly needed to feed billions of people around the globe and provide nutrition for the animals we eat.

Grains have become very easy to transport, are fast to cook, easy to chew, and easily digested and absorbed (except by people with celiac disease or grain allergies). Milling grains to create flour makes them easy to store without refrigeration. Advances in refining can produce starches and flours with qualities that chefs can exploit to create a multitude of dishes and products. For example, wheat can be refined into flour with a high protein content to make crusty or chewy breads, or low protein content suitable for cakes, cookies, and piecrusts. Wheat flour is commonly used to thicken gravy and sauces. The variety of edible products that can be made with carbohydrates from grains is never-ending, and these food items tempt people throughout the world.

Carbohydrate intake from grains now accounts for over 50 percent of the daily calories in the typical adult diet in the US. Even the USDA recommends multiple servings of grains per day. Many expert panels encourage the consumption of "whole grain" products, believing in their health benefits just because they contain B vitamins, vitamin E, and fiber normally associated with bran. The medical community further aids this myth with pronouncements exalting the virtues of eating the first meal of the day in the form of usually some grain-based cereal, oatmeal, or bread that gets you ready for school, work, or other activities. They emphasize this directive by warning that those who don't eat breakfast are likely to consume a mid-morning snack containing more calories than they would have consumed at breakfast.

The food industry has been happy to exploit this opportunity by marketing easy-to-prepare cereals and many grain-based products for breakfast. Food companies even procure endorsements from medical associations and experts regarding products made with whole grains. They promote the virtues of the vitamins, minerals, and proteins they have added to grain-based products, or the deletion of particles such as gluten from these products. Focusing on these supposed health benefits in their advertising has made it easier for the general population to completely overlook the serious impact that the carbs in grains and grain-based foods have on their blood glucose levels.

Is there any proof of this theory?

In my view, there is very strong evidence in the fact that everywhere in the world where grains have become or are becoming an increasing staple of the diet, we see a fast-rising incidence of Type 2 diabetes. Consider these two specific studies.

American Indians. The prevalence of Type 2 diabetes among 2917 Pima Indians over age 35 living in Arizona who were studied between 1965 and 1969 was nearly 50% of the population, the highest incidence of diabetes among a distinct group of people ever recorded, as reported in July 1971 in the medical journal, *The Lancet.* This was not an isolated finding. More than 30% of people aged 25 and over among other Native American tribes — the Seneca, Cherokee, and Cocopah — also had Type 2 diabetes. Although the researchers concluded, "The reasons for such a high frequency of diabetes mellitus are obscure," they speculated that there was a strong possible connection between the tribes' obesity and diabetes and the altering of their traditional diet to the typical American diet after the tribes were confined to reservations. Like many Indian tribes, the Pima had made a profound change in what they ate, and the consequence was their shockingly high incidence of diabetes.

When American Indian tribes were living in their natural environments on the plains, their diet consisted largely of vegetables, fruits, nuts, eggs, fish, and meat from animals they hunted. But when Indians were confined to reservations, their meals switched to contain substantially more grain-based foods, amounting to as much as

50% of their total dietary energy intake. The link between this radical change in diet for an entire culture residing in different locations and the resulting alarmingly high incidence of diabetes cannot be a coincidence.

In fact, according to the National Indian Council on Aging, in 2019, American Indians and Alaska Natives had the highest diabetes prevalence rates of all racial and ethnic groups in the United States. The US Centers for Disease Control and Prevention (CDC) predicted that one in two American Indian and Alaska Native children born in 2000 will have Type 2 diabetes in their lifetime unless the current trend is halted.

Australian Aborigines. Another fascinating study that supports the impact of grains in causing Type 2 diabetes was done in Australia. In the 1970s, researcher Kerin O'Dea persuaded ten (five men and five women) fully diabetic Australian Aborigines with an average age of 54 to give up their urban diet and spend 7 weeks living as hunter-gatherers in their traditional country in northwestern Australia. In the wild, they ate kangaroo meat, turtle, crocodile, fish, wild yams, and other foods, like their forefathers had. While their urban diet had consisted of about 50% carbohydrates (from flour, rice, potatoes, sugared drinks, and alcohol), 40% fat from meat, and 10% protein, their diet in the wild averaged 61% protein, 24% fat, and only 16% carbohydrate. The results of this 7-week experiment showed that every single participant had lowered their blood sugar to normal levels.

While the researchers conducting this experiment believed that the reduced blood sugar levels were the result of the low-fat diet, I suggest that this experiment is yet another definitive proof that it is the reduction in carbohydrate consumption that led to lower blood sugar — in as little as 7 weeks. Dropping from 50% carbohydrate to just 16% carbohydrate in one's diet is a much more significant change than that in fat intake. While many researchers in the 1970s were focused on the role of fat in causing heart disease, and rightfully so, we now know that the real source of that fat was the liver manufacturing it from excess glucose absorbed from the gut.

These two studies, though done on different people at different times, function together in a scientific way to help us see the link between grains and diabetes. Establishing cause and effect is a universally accepted method of validating a scientific concept. In both of these studies, it seems clear that a diet high in carbohydrates can be linked directly to Type 2 diabetes. Introducing grain-based foods into the environment of Native American tribes resulted in significant incidence of Type 2 diabetes. Removing grains, the same agent, from the environment of the Australian Aborigines showed significant reversal of Type 2 diabetes.

In my opinion, there should no longer be any doubt as to the cause — the overconsumption of grain-based foods — and the effect — Type 2 diabetes. World cereal production went from 2.82 billion metric tons in 2014 to 3.07 billion in 2021 as reported by the World Bank, as the global population increased from 7.318 billion in 2014 to 7.888 billion in 2021.

There are differences in the amount of grain consumed in different parts of the world. For example, the proportion of total energy provided by carbohydrates in the diet is roughly 70% or more in Asia and Africa, while the percentage of energy from carbohydrates is only about 50% in the developed world where people have a higher intake of protein and fat.

However, both levels of grain consumption are too high for good health. In a finding reported in *The Lancet Oncology* in 2002, it was stated that, over the past few decades, the proportion of people with excess body weight had been increasing in both the developed and developing nations. In 2021, the World Health Organization reported that worldwide obesity has tripled since 1975.[2]

The conclusion I draw from analyzing these studies is that the increasingly common incidence of diabetes (and obesity) in many nations of Western Europe and in India, China, and many other Asian countries can only be correlated with the intake of grains and grain-flour products.

A Mistaken Science Led Us in the Wrong Direction

In the US, one of the major factors behind our love for grains arose out of a misguided war against fat. In the mid-1980s, a million Americans were dying from heart disease, believed to be caused by the consumption of fatty foods. Several scientists published articles with research that showed that fat—specifically low-density lipoprotein (LDL) cholesterol—clogs arteries. Politicians influenced by those reports declared war on fat. The US National Institutes of Health recommended that all Americans eat less fat and cholesterol to reduce the risk of heart disease.

In response, the food industry began promulgating the virtues of "healthy" carbohydrates over fats. Americans bought into that marketing and increased their intake of carbohydrates while reducing their consumption of fat. Grain-based cereals for breakfast, sandwiches for lunch, and starches (rice, potatoes, or corn) to accompany dinners became staples of the American diet, along with mass-produced donuts, cakes, pies, pasta, pizza, and breads. The result: the noted medical journal, *Lancet Oncology,* stated in 2021 that the prevalence of Type 2 diabetes among adults increased over 250% from 1980 to 2021.

Our unthinking attitude about grains

Today, most people accept grains as if they are a required part of their daily diet. Generations of people have grown up with grains and cannot imagine eating a meal without bread, potatoes, rice, or corn.

Although statistics prove that the more grains people eat, the higher the incidence of Type 2 diabetes, most people (and doctors) have a cavalier attitude about grains. This gives food manufacturers and marketers ammunition to entice us to consume more and more grain-based foods. In our globalized world, it is easy to find grain products like these everywhere: bagels, baguettes, breadsticks, buns, croissants, pretzels, and rolls; challah, chapatti, focaccia, injera, lavash, naan, paratha, roti, pita, pizza, and tortilla; bhatura, frybread, puri, and sopaipilla; biscuits, cakes, crackers, cupcakes, doughnuts, muffins, and pastries; mantou, pot stickers, dumplings, noodles, and other pastas; crepes, pancakes, pies, and other food products prepared with grain flours using ethnic cuisines and regional flavors.

These all sound so good, don't they? But eating them puts you at risk of high blood sugar and eventually diabetes.

So what exactly is the link between grains and diabetes? Why do you need to reduce your grain consumption to as low as possible? How does not eating grains help you reverse your diabetes? Read on.

CHAPTER 2

THE OLD THEORIES ABOUT THE CAUSE OF DIABETES

THERE ARE two common explanations — "insulin deficiency" or "insulin resistance" — for why people develop Type 2 diabetes.

Neither explanation specifically blames grains as the cause, and thus both miss the clear link between the enormous percentage of grain-based foods in our diet and the rising incidence of Type 2 diabetes in nations throughout the world. Neither explanation can account for many inconsistencies in understanding why people develop high blood sugar and end up with diabetes — precisely because these explanations do not recognize the triggering role that grains play in altering the biology of the body.

Let's look at these two explanations and you will see why I consider them incorrect, and why the explanation that I provide to you afterwards makes far more biological and logical sense — and points to the cure that allows you to reverse your diabetes.

The dysfunctional pancreas theory

This theory is the earliest explanation for why adults develop Type 2 diabetes. It was based on tests that showed that diabetics can have high blood sugar but low insulin levels in the blood. A normal body metabolism should call for more insulin to be released from the pancreas as blood glucose levels rise after a carbohydrate-rich meal. The suspicion was therefore that the insulin-response system in the pancreas is dysfunctional. This defect effectively causes the pancreas to not release an adequate supply of insulin relative to the amount of glucose entering the bloodstream from the intestine. Over time, the theory contends, you end up with a constant state of high blood sugar and diabetes, requiring insulin injections to supplement the dysfunctional pancreas.

What's wrong with the dysfunctional pancreas theory?

First, this theory has not been proven. No gene mutation has been found to explain why a dysfunctional pancreas develops or affects only some people. No explanation has been found for why this same dysfunction occurs in an overweight person, a lean person, and a pregnant woman who develops diabetes. Nor is there an explanation for how the pancreas can suddenly regain its functionality when an obese person loses weight or after the birth of the child in a pregnant diabetic. In addition, no one has demonstrated a faulty mechanism responsible for reducing the secretion of insulin from the pancreas when there is glucose in the blood. There is also the question: Is the reason or the mechanism of the supposed insufficient insulin release the same among all these people? If so, that seems strange. If not, on what basis can experts claim that different reasons produce the same functional defect in the same organ, the pancreas? Is there possibly another cause for high blood sugar among these three very different types of people?

The theory also fails to recognize a basic biological fact— the brain regulates the release of hormones in the body. In fact, the minute-by-minute adjustments that keep one's blood glucose level normal involve the combined actions of insulin plus three other hormones— glucagon, epinephrine, and cortisol. The brain integrates this process to control the release of all four hormones. This means that claiming that only pancreatic cells become dysfunctional while the other three hormone-release mechanisms behave normally is illogical.

The role of the brain in regulating hormones provides the most logical explanation for why diabetics may have high blood sugar and low levels of insulin. When blood sugar rises, it sends a strong signal to the pancreas to release insulin. However, in people whose diet creates a continuously high level of blood sugar, the brain's control center eventually sends a signal to the pancreas to reduce the release of insulin in order to preserve the functionality of the insulin-producing pancreatic cells as well as to protect the body from undesired effects of the hormone.

There is a good reason for the brain to assert this control. Insulin not only signals cells to absorb glucose, but it also influences the metabolism of fatty acids and amino acids, acid secretion in the stomach, sodium excretion in the kidney, and other biological activities in the body. In addition, insulin acts as a "growth" hormone, promoting cells to divide. Too much insulin results in excessive cell divisions. This is why diabetics have higher rates of cancers of the pancreas, liver, colorectum, breast, urinary tract, and endometrium than people who do not have diabetes. In effect, the brain intentionally aims to curtail insulin release despite continuously long periods of high blood sugar.

Ultimately, the pancreas dysfunction theory makes little biological sense and remains unproven, despite decades of research. If anything, the pancreas is producing insulin, but not enough because the person is consuming a consistently high carbohydrate diet. It is not that the pancreas is dysfunctional; it is simply overloaded. This explanation supports my theory that diet is the cause of Type 2 diabetes, along with the role played by the fatty acid burn switch.

The insulin resistance theory

The insulin resistance theory is the dominant explanation for the cause of Type 2 diabetes. According to this theory, for some reason, the body's cells become "insensitive" and do not respond to the insulin hormone. This causes glucose to remain in the bloodstream rather than entering cells, even when there are adequate levels of insulin in the blood.

Why does this happen? Oddly enough, medical science has not yet been able to explain why this supposed insulin resistance occurs, nor by exactly what biological mechanism it happens. It remains unexplained why billions of cells suddenly switch to resist the presence of insulin to allow glucose to enter them when those cells didn't have the problem before.

One of the most suspicious (and biologically illogical) elements of this theory is that insulin resistance does not occur in all the body's cells. There are 200 types of cells in the body, but the theory states that insulin resistance occurs in only three main groups of cells:

1. muscle cells that have not been warmed up (inactive muscle cells),
2. the liver, and
3. fat cells.

No matter how much biological science you know or don't know, it is clear this theory does not make sense. Why would only three types of cells become resistant to insulin?

Let's look at each of these types:

Muscle cells — It is known that active, exercising muscle does not need the assistance of insulin to let glucose enter the cells. However, when muscle cells have been resting, the insulin resistance theory claims that there is a sharp reduction in the amount of glucose that diffuses into the cells, despite the presence of insulin outside. This is considered evidence that the muscle cells are "resisting" the action of insulin through some type of faulty internal mechanism.

Liver cells — It is also thought that the liver becomes resistant to insulin because in Type 2 diabetes, the liver continues to release glucose even when the bloodstream is already overflowing with it and insulin is present in an adequate amount. Normally, insulin would block the liver from releasing glucose. Thus, it is theorized that liver cells also become resistant to insulin's effects.

Fat cells — You need to know a bit of biology to understand why the insulin resistance theory believes that fat cells can become resistant to insulin. Normally, after meals, digestion produces glucose from the foods you have eaten. In about four hours after the meal, glucose molecules not picked up by cells in the body are converted in the liver first to fatty acids and then to fat called triglycerides. The blood then takes these triglycerides to fat tissue for storage.

But the triglyceride molecule is too large to enter the fat cell. The role of insulin here is to activate an enzyme called *lipase* outside the fat cell that tells it to break down the triglyceride molecules back into small fatty acids that can go through the fat cell membrane. Once inside, three fatty acids recombine with a molecule of glycerol manufactured from glucose inside the fat cell (hence the name triglyceride) for storage.

Triglyceride produced in the liver arriving at a fat cell is too large to enter. Insulin activates external lipase outside the fat cell to break the triglyceride molecules into fatty acids that can enter the cell. Inside, these fatty acids are reconstituted into triglyceride for storage.

Whenever your body needs extra energy, another lipase enzyme *inside* the fat cell breaks the stored triglycerides back down into fatty acids that can exit out of the fat cell into the bloodstream. These fatty acids then flow to wherever the body needs them, such as muscle cells that can extract energy from fatty acids, just as they can from glucose. Ordinarily, the presence of insulin outside the fat cell inhibits this interior lipase enzyme from releasing fatty acids from stored triglyceride.

Normally the presence of insulin prevents internal lipase from releasing fatty acids from triglycerides.

However, according to the insulin resistance theory, it is thought that something goes wrong with this process. In diabetics, large amounts of fatty acids are released from fat tissue, even in the presence of insulin. This supposedly explains why people with Type 2 diabetes have high levels of fatty acids in their blood.

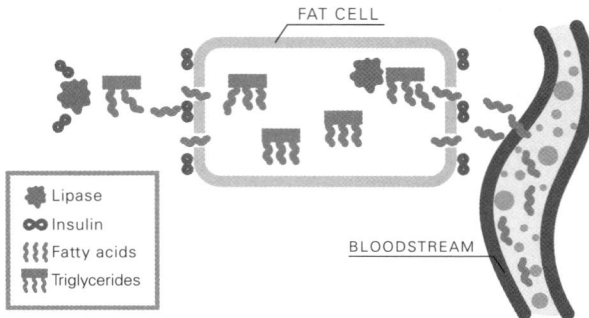

The insulin resistance theory claims that insulin triggers external lipase (left) to break down triglycerides into fatty acids that can enter the fat cell. But the theory also claims that internal lipase is resistant to insulin and so it allows fatty acids to exit the fat cell and go into the bloodstream, even when insulin is present.

What's wrong with the insulin resistance theory?

Frankly, a lot. I have examined the insulin resistance theory in depth for more than 25 years, and it is demonstrably flawed. It has also never been shown in a scientific way why resistance to insulin starts or what biological mechanism in a cell could possibly cause such resistance. Here are some specific arguments about why the insulin resistance theory is illogical.

1. *It is not logical that millions of people around the world are evolving to have resistance to a natural body hormone.*

   As mentioned, the incidence of diabetes is increasing in every nation in the world where grains are becoming a major portion of the diet. It does not make sense that some humans, but not all, in these countries are evolving in a very short time to be resistant to a natural body hormone that helps them utilize glucose as fuel for energy. Diabetes is not a contagious disease, and no other hormones are being affected to the extent that we see among the increasing numbers of people developing Type 2 diabetes.

2. *It is not logical that only 3 types of cells develop resistance.*

   There are over 200 types of cells in the body, so it should be argued that every one of them should develop insulin resistance at the same time. But the theory does not explain why this does not occur. Meanwhile, no one has proposed a theory that explains how cells other than these three avoid the fate of becoming resistant to the action of insulin.

3. *The way insulin resistance affects cells is inconsistent.*

   I discussed above that when triglycerides arrive at fat cells to be stored, they are broken down into fatty acids that can pass through the fat cell membrane, while inside the fat cell, the fatty acids are recombined back into triglycerides. Both actions are triggered by an enzyme called lipase that resides outside and inside the fat cells. But there is an illogical element of the insulin resistance theory here: it claims that insulin resistance affects the *internal* lipase but not the *external* lipase. The two enzymes are exactly the same, so how could opposite responses occur to them?

4.   *There is no loss of the body's ability to regulate heat.*

If the millions of cells in the body were resistant to insulin, and thus not getting glucose for their energy production, particularly in our muscle tissue, we would expect the body to have great difficulty regulating its consistent internal temperature, 98.6 degrees Fahrenheit. The body is like a home furnace that burns glucose to produce heat. Under normal conditions, the temperature of the inner core of the human body remains constant within ±1 degree Fahrenheit 24 hours a day. Even when the outside air temperature ranges from a low of 55 degrees Fahrenheit below zero to a high of 130 degrees Fahrenheit, the body still maintains an almost constant internal core body temperature, even if our skin temperature rises and falls with the temperature of the surroundings.

So the question is: if your cells, especially muscle cells, are insulin resistant and not receiving glucose to create both energy and heat for your body, then how can the body maintain its core temperature? The fact is, there is no evidence that diabetics have body temperature maintenance problems, another sign that the insulin resistance theory is illogical.

5.   *There is no loss of muscle strength in diabetics.*

Similar to the body heat counterargument against the insulin resistance theory, we should also question why the body does not lose muscular strength. If insulin resistance prevents muscles from using glucose, why don't we see evidence of diabetics having weakening muscle function, just as you would expect an automobile to function poorly if the engine's ability to burn gasoline was impaired? But in fact, Type 2 diabetes does not prevent people from running, jumping, lifting heavy boxes, dancing, skiing, or walking.

Type 2 diabetics are often aging seniors who are losing muscle mass, but not at rates faster than the general population of seniors who do not have diabetes. There is no evidence of progressive weakening of muscle power or deterioration of muscle function in individuals with decades-long Type 2 diabetes, even if they require increasing doses of medications including insulin to regulate their blood sugar levels. In short, it seems unlikely that insulin resistance prevents muscles from obtaining energy, even if it is not facilitating the entry of glucose.

6. *There is no finding of any agents that block insulin or proof of cellular changes.*

No research has discovered or demonstrated an actual agent that blocks the binding of insulin with the insulin receptor on cells at the time Type 2 diabetes is diagnosed. In contrast, with many diseases, an agent such as an antibody has been found to be responsible for blocking the response by cells in the body.

Similarly, there is no proof of any type of change in cells that might make them suddenly resist insulin. Research has not identified any differences in cells that are supposedly insulin resistant and those that are not.

7. *Short-term diabetes in pregnant women is strong proof against the insulin resistance theory.*

Gestational diabetes mellitus (GDM) is a condition that affects almost 10% of pregnancies in Western countries. It is usually diagnosed between weeks 12–16 of pregnancy, and, oddly, it almost always disappears within days following delivery.

Why do some women get GDM? It is generally believed that the cause is the same as Type 2 diabetes — insulin resistance. How does that happen? Scientists claim the placenta is responsible for triggering or significantly worsening insulin insensitivity in the three cell types. As to why it disappears rapidly after delivery, the argument is that eliminating the placenta changes the conditions.

But is this logical, I ask? Given that men and non-pregnant women usually take years to develop high blood sugar and eventually diabetes, how is it possible that a pregnant woman can develop diabetes within 12–16 weeks? If each cell is an independent body, how do billions of cells suddenly convert to being insulin resistant within this short period of time — and then flip flop back to being insulin sensitive only days after birth?

Secondly, with over 200 types of cells in the human body, why and how do "messengers" from the placenta zero in on the same three types of cells (muscle cells, liver, and fat) as in Type 2 diabetes, to tell them to resist insulin? How do those three types of cells decipher the message to make them insensitive only to insulin and not to other hormones in the body?

And finally, given that 40% of mothers who developed gestational diabetes end up developing Type 2 diabetes within the ten subsequent years after giving birth, this suggests that factors other than the presence of the placenta are responsible for the development of GDM.

———

Some researchers, medical practitioners, and diabetes educators, finding it difficult to let go of a theory they have been working with for a long time, demand experimental proof for the absence of insulin resistance, instead of their own asking for or providing proof of its existence. The fact remains that even 80 years after widespread acceptance of the insulin resistance theory, no one has explained whether the mechanism is the same in all three sites purported to be having it.

In addition, the ability to measure the degree of resistance is lacking. If it were known, it could lead to targeted therapy based on the site and degree of resistance. But currently, medical practitioners prescribe the same medication, insulin, to which the patient is supposedly resistant, to force muscles to accept *more* glucose and the liver to release *less*, without any way to measure the success of insulin to reduce the resistance in any of the sites. Contrast this illogical procedure with the common medical practice whereby doctors stop giving an antibiotic or chemo agent to a patient who has developed resistance to it.

Some researchers have sought to provide an explanation for the development of insulin resistance by correlating it with the intake of foods containing high fructose corn syrup. This ignores the more obvious elephant in the room — enormous amounts of glucose molecules absorbed from grain-based carbohydrate by the same individual. Still others talk about insulin resistance caused by environmental agents entering the body and/or imbalance in intestinal organisms, yet they cannot explain how high blood sugar can become reversed after weight loss following delivery in a pregnant diabetic or after bariatric surgery in an obese diabetic.

The only logical conclusion: insulin resistance is incorrect

Taken together, these arguments point to gaping holes in the theory of insulin resistance as the cause of Type 2 diabetes. To date, there is absolutely no proof that insulin resistance accurately explains why the body's cells do not intake glucose the way they normally do.

Furthermore, we have no information on the reason why or the mechanism by which cells suddenly become resistant. Nor do we have a test to measure the degree of insulin resistance among any of these cells, which could facilitate the development of targeted treatment of diabetes specific to the site and severity of resistance. Based on the above arguments, it is scientifically unsound to claim that Type 2 diabetes is caused by insulin resistance.

Why the cause of diabetes matters to you?

The discussion in this chapter negating the two common theories as the cause of diabetes is vital to you. This is not purely an intellectual exercise comparing three competing theories. So which of these theories makes more sense?

1. Your eating habits or some other factor causes dysfunction of your pancreas to produce too little insulin;
2. Your genes or some other mechanism causes three types of cells in your body to become insulin resistant; or
3. The cause of high blood sugar and diabetes, as I have suggested, is the consumption of grains.

Understanding which of these three possibilities is the TRUE cause of high blood sugar can make a real difference in how you and your doctor decide to help you reverse your diabetes.

For instance, if you believe in the genetic cause, you might feel helpless if you think you already have genes that are responsible for your Type 2 diabetes. You may give up hope of ever reversing it, accepting your diabetes as an inevitable long-term disease you will carry for the rest of your life, requiring medication and possibly insulin injections.

Let me correct this impression though. No one has identified specific genes responsible for Type 2 diabetes. Whatever genes you have, you had them from day one of your life, yet diabetes did not appear in your infancy.

Or you may believe (and your doctor may tell you) that weight gain caused your cells to become resistant to insulin. However, as I described above, the mechanism for this scenario has never been explained. In addition, if weight gain is responsible for causing insulin resistance, why does diabetes occur in thin people? Moreover, if something other than weight gain is responsible for the appearance of diabetes in lean people, why does it not happen from day one of their lives since they had the same genes at that time.

Or if you believe your eating habits are responsible for causing a dysfunctional pancreas, you still may not know the precise nature of what is wrong in your diet, what food choice changes are necessary and, most importantly, how this change can be achieved. You may also be confused because Type 2 diabetes is appearing with increased frequency in India, China, and the United States — countries with very different cuisines and eating habits. Some proponents of the insulin resistance theory blame chemicals such as pesticides incorporated into the food chain. However, until a definite cause and effect is established, this explanation is still just speculation.

Finally, maybe your attitude is, "It doesn't matter what the cause is, I can live with it because I can just take a pill," or, if your blood sugar remains consistently very high, you might think, "I'll just give myself insulin injections whenever I need to."

These are both very dangerous conclusions. Believe me, they are a slippery slope — because it is well known that people who start out on low dosages of a diabetes medication often end up increasing that dosage, changing to a different or combination of medications, and finally injecting insulin, or taking medications that cause release of insulin from their own pancreas.

I want to tell you that this is not how you want to live, your days dictated by medication and feeding schedules. Today's medical profession has a propensity to jump quickly to treating all illnesses and conditions with medications. Meanwhile, the pharmaceutical industry seems to have no problem considering all diseases as long-term conditions for which they can sell you drugs. As an MD, I am not averse to medications, but they should be used as sparingly as possible, and only when necessary.

According to my theory about consuming grains as the cause of diabetes, you will learn that some simple and easy-to-implement lifestyle changes can literally lower your blood sugar, regardless of your body weight, and that diabetes is not as irreversible a disease as it is made out to be. By understanding the real cause of it, you can truly reverse it. Let me give you a clue: the sugar that appears in your blood has to enter the body through your mouth. What you eat is what causes high blood sugar. It's really no surprise.

A MORE LOGICAL THEORY TO EXPLAIN WHY YOU HAVE TYPE 2 DIABETES

I F THE DYSFUNCTIONAL pancreas theory and the insulin resistance theory are not accurate, what could possibly explain why some people develop Type 2 diabetes?

I believe I have uncovered the most logical and biologically consistent answer. As mentioned, this new explanation reveals the strong link between the consumption of grains, high blood sugar, and diabetes. This theory explains why younger and younger children are developing diabetes, why pregnant women can develop gestational diabetes and quickly lose it after giving birth, and why thin people can also end up with diabetes. Overall, my explanation for the cause of high blood sugar and diabetes can account for many of the biological inconsistencies that occur if we continue to blindly accept either the dysfunctional pancreas theory or the insulin resistance theory.

Explaining the real reason why you have high blood sugar and develop diabetes — and how grains are a direct cause of these conditions — requires a small amount of science education. Although you may not have had a biology class in decades, or you simply don't enjoy reading science, I encourage you to give the following section a try. I have kept it as simple as possible, so that the average non-scientist can understand it. The more you follow this explanation, the more convinced you will become that you can control your own health and reverse your diabetes.

The real cause of high blood sugar

The actual trigger of high blood sugar that leads to diabetes does indeed have to do with the consumption of grains and grain-flour products. I am referring to wheat, oats, barley, rye, corn, rice, and other common grains. It is not that these grains trigger insulin resistance in any cell in the body or wear out the insulin-producing cells in your pancreas to cause the initiation of high blood sugar. It is rather that the continual consumption of grains and grain-flour products overwhelms the body's normal metabolism related to carbohydrate-rich foods and glucose.

To explain this process, I will enumerate a sequence of events that over time cause high blood sugar and diabetes.

These first six steps explain what happens to nutrients absorbed after a meal.

1. First, it is important to understand that everything you eat that contains *complex carbohydrates* — such as bread, croissants, muffins, sweet rolls, rice, pizza dough — break down in the small intestine first to *maltose*, and then to the most basic form of carbohydrate, called *glucose*. Dairy products like milk and yogurt have a form of sugar called *lactose,* and this, too, may eventually be changed into glucose. Fruits contain a natural sugar, *sucrose,* which may also be broken down into glucose. The rest of the foods you eat break down into fatty acids, amino acids, cholesterol, minerals, vitamins, and many other

micronutrients that the cells of your body need to function. All the absorbed nutrients enter the general blood circulation for a journey to the millions of cells in your body.

2. As nutrient absorption into your bloodstream continues, all the carbohydrates that have ultimately broken down into glucose cause your 'blood sugar' level to climb. This stimulates your pancreas to release insulin that informs cells about the presence of glucose outside the cell membrane, triggering cells to absorb that glucose. This action feeds your cells, especially muscle cells that burn the glucose to create the energy they need to function.

3. Glucose also arrives in your liver, which converts some of it into glycogen and keeps it in storage. Between meals, when your body needs more energy than that already existing in the cells, the liver breaks the glycogen back down again into glucose and ships it out to the bloodstream on a fairly regular basis in an effort to maintain a constant blood sugar level. Insulin plays a role in this process by preventing the liver from breaking down glycogen when there is already sufficient glucose in your bloodstream.

4. Any remaining excess glucose in your blood is converted to fatty acids by the liver. The liver uses these fatty acids along with the other fatty acids from the food you eat, to manufacture *triglycerides*. The liver sends these triglycerides to the fat cells in your tummy, thighs, buttocks, and many other places of the body for storage. When your body needs more fuel than the available glucose, the triglycerides are broken back down into fatty acids that enter the bloodstream and flow throughout the body to cells that need them. *This is because your body's cells are like a hybrid car that can burn either glucose or fatty acids.* This is a normal body metabolism (see sidebar on how your muscle cells burn both glucose and fatty acids).

Muscle cells burn both glucose and fatty acids for energy

Muscle cells (which are the largest user of glucose in the body) can produce energy in two ways.

The first step in converting glucose into ATP is the process called *glycolysis.* This is done outside the cell's mitochondria and oxygen is not required. Muscle cells do this for about the first 10 seconds of activity.

The second is by burning glucose or fatty acids inside the mitochondria, a process that requires oxygen. When more energy is needed after those first 10 seconds, muscle cells will switch to burning fatty acids inside the mitochondria, because when it comes to muscle energy production, glucose was simply a "starter." *When your body has fatty acids in the bloodstream and a large storage of triglycerides in your fat cells, this switch to burning fatty acids on a consistent basis is what I believe is the cause of Type 2 diabetes, as it leaves glucose in the bloodstream, thus high blood sugar.*

Given that humans are built to store only a small amount (120 grams) of glucose in the liver, this suggests that nature never intended humans to use glucose as our primary method of fueling our muscle cells. However, glucose is used for the initial construction of cells (because when no functional mitochondria yet exists, it is not possible for the cell to burn fatty acids). Glucose is also the primary fuel for nerve cells, including brain cells. But it appears that nature intended human muscle cells to burn fatty acids, not glucose, for the majority of their energy production. Otherwise one would have expected facilities for easier transport of glucose, such as those found in nerve cells, to be also present in muscle fibers, but they are not.

5.   When people overconsume grains at meals, they produce large amounts of glucose beyond what the body can use on an immediate basis. Especially if you are inactive, much of the glucose in the liver is converted to triglycerides and sent to your fat cells for storage. As you might imagine, the consistent overconsumption of grains leads to adding more and more storage in your fat cells, creating weight gain. The overconsumption of any food contributes to weight gain as well, because your body's total weight is made up from the combination of your bones, organs, tissues, fat cells, and blood. But overall, in today's lifestyle, grains and grain-flour products are the main culprits in building up your body's storage of fat, irrespective of where you live.

6.   Each person has a genetically determined allocation of fat cells and stem cells that can become fat cells in the body. Some people have very few fat cells while others have large numbers of them, a function of their genetic inheritance directly from their parents, as well as from their long-term ethnic heritage generations before their parents. In the same way that some people are tall and others are short, and two siblings born to the same parents can grow to different heights, some people are naturally thin, while others are chunky or fat, even within the same family. The overconsumption of food, particularly grains, can cause even thin people to gain weight, although they may not show it in terms of looking fatter to others because they simply have fewer fat cells. Weight tables and other charts that are used for classification may falsely reassure people that their body weight is acceptable, even when their allotted fat cells are filled to capacity, while excess fat stays in their blood and tissues.

These next steps explain how high blood sugar occurs, leading to diabetes.

7.   Given that people have only a certain allocation of fat cells, whatever their body type, what happens when their fat cells

become full and there is nowhere for the excess glucose they produce from overconsuming grains to go? This is precisely where a normal body metabolism sets off a chain reaction that leads to high blood sugar. It begins when the liver sends triglycerides to fat cells for storage. But triglyceride molecules are too big to enter the walls of fat cells, so a protein called *lipase* breaks them down into fatty acids that enter the fat cells, where they are reconstituted into triglycerides for storage. However, when your fat cells are full, those fatty acids cannot enter, and they remain in the blood stream.

8. It is at this point that you begin to be at risk for high blood sugar. When you continue to overeat or become less active, and you fill your fat cells, you end up causing your bloodstream to become filled with fatty acids that have nowhere to be stored. As mentioned above, your body's cells can burn glucose or fatty acids to fuel their energy needs. Generally, glucose is utilized first, but when fatty acids are readily available, cells will begin using them first. Why?

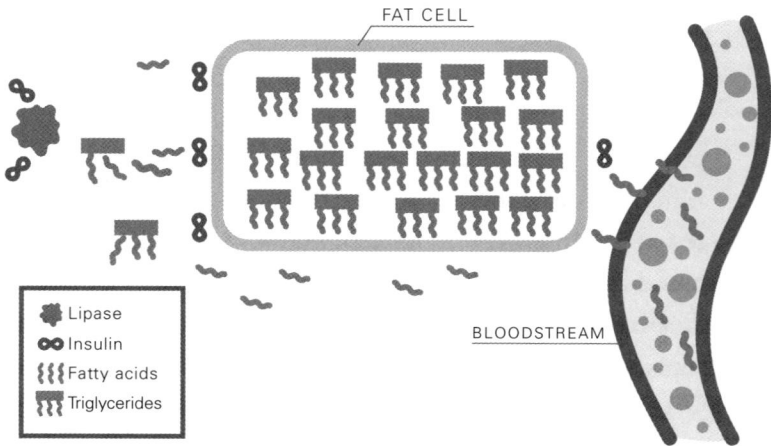

My theory shows how fatty acids released outside the fat cell by the external lipase in the presence of insulin are not welcome inside because the cell is already filled with triglycerides. These fatty acids therefore enter the bloodstream.

The main reason is that fatty acids are made of the same molecules as the membrane of cells. This means that fatty acids slip right into cells, whereas glucose needs help from transporters inside the cell and, often, the presence of insulin outside to enter the cell.

9. When you have filled your fat cells, causing your bloodstream to overflow with fatty acids, you create the conditions for muscle cells to begin burning fatty acids on a regular basis. What is actually happening is that your muscle cells are not resistant to insulin at all. They simply don't need any glucose because they have plenty of fatty acids to burn. And because your muscles, on average, constitute about 40% of body mass, their activity accounts for much of the body's energy expenditure. For example, even at rest, skeletal muscles use energy to maintain their normal metabolic activities at a rate of three times that of fat tissue of comparable weight. This means that, in general, your body as a whole is burning more fatty acids than glucose for energy production.

Muscle cells can burn glucose or fatty acids. The abundance of fatty acids in your blood triggers muscle cells to begin burning fatty acids rather than glucose. Once muscle cells have switched to burning fatty acids, even the presence of insulin cannot force glucose into the cells since they simply don't need it. As a result, glucose remains in your bloodstream, causing high blood sugar.

The fatty acid burn switch

The steps I described above fully explain why the overconsumption of grains causes weight gain and high blood sugar, often leading to Type 2 diabetes. I call my theory about this cause of diabetes "the fatty acid burn switch" because, as mentioned, high blood sugar is triggered not by insulin resistance but rather by filling your fat cells and causing large amounts of fatty acids to flow through your bloodstream, which causes your muscle cells to switch to burning fatty acids rather than glucose. The result is that glucose remains unused in your bloodstream, hence high blood sugar.

One irrefutable proof of my theory is that people with high blood sugar and diabetes have not just high levels of glucose in their blood, but high levels of triglycerides and fatty acids. Interestingly, the levels of triglycerides and fatty acids in the blood of people who overeat could be higher long before their blood glucose level starts a steady upward climb towards diabetes.[3]

It has even been known for more than 30 years that most patients with Type 2 diabetes have elevated fatty acid levels. In 1994, the *Journal of Clinical Investigation* reported that skeletal muscles have impaired glucose uptake and utilization directly proportional to the elevation of blood fatty acid concentration even in the presence of insulin. This finding was misinterpreted though as being due to insulin resistance, rather than as my theory suggests, the normal body metabolism that muscle cells will burn primarily fatty acids rather than glucose when there is an abundance of fatty acids in the bloodstream.

Is the switch permanent?

Muscle cells do not necessarily switch to burning fatty acids rather than glucose on a permanent basis. They burn whatever is most immediately available. But if your blood contains high levels of fatty acids that slip through the cell membranes without difficulty, they become the fuel most frequently utilized. In fact, muscle cells can and do utilize large amounts of fatty acids to produce energy on a daily basis, but with diabetes, they are using fatty acids nearly all the time, leaving glucose in the bloodstream.

What's important to keep in mind about my alternate explanation of the cause of Type 2 diabetes is that it points to a logical natural cause — too much fat being stored in your body. Since your fat cells are full, they are unable to accept more fatty acids, which then circulate in the bloodstream and become the fuel of choice for your muscles.

This suggests that there is a natural antidote to lowering blood sugar and reversing diabetes — *stop consuming grains!* A diet that substantially reduces grain consumption as much as possible will help you empty your fat cells, which can eventually lead to helping your muscle cells revert to burning glucose again.

Why does the body allow high blood sugar to happen?

If you are wondering why the body allows this switch to burning fatty acids to occur, there is a good reason related to self-preservation, as in many metabolic processes. In this case, when your blood glucose level starts an upward climb, the pancreas, as programmed, releases more insulin to keep the glucose level within the optimal range for your body. Insulin accomplishes this by instructing the liver to convert all the excess glucose into fatty acids and triglycerides. The body expects to be able to store this excess in its fat cells.

However, as your blood sugar level keeps climbing because of the lack of storage capacity, the control centers in the brain must decide whether to continue releasing more and more insulin to moderate the blood glucose level, or to tolerate a higher circulating level of glucose to preserve the long-term health of your pancreas.

In the end, the brain opts for a balanced approach. It allows for the elevation of blood sugar, knowing that it can get rid of the glucose through urination once the level reaches above 180 mg/dl. This helps preserve the functional life of pancreatic cells in charge of secreting insulin. In addition, the control center may be trying to prevent undesirable side effects of excess insulin such as stimulation of cancer cell growth and development of polycystic ovary syndrome.

Begin tracking your blood triglyceride counts

If you have not yet been diagnosed with diabetes, ask your doctor to begin tracking your blood triglyceride levels. If you are overeating and your fat cells are filling up, the triglycerides that your liver produces from the carbohydrate and fat in your food cannot be stored. Triglycerides, not being water soluble, cannot be excreted in your urine and therefore remain in your body. Thus, noting a rise in your triglycerides over time suggests you may be at risk for diabetes.

Ideally, your triglyceride count should remain below 150 mg/dl if you want to stay below the risk level for high blood sugar. Ask your doctor to review your blood triglyceride count over the past years of blood tests and continue to track it in the future. If you detect a rising pattern, stop eating grains to lose weight as soon as possible. This will prevent the switch in fuels from occurring.

ONLY THE "FATTY ACID BURN THEORY" CAN EXPLAIN THE INCONSISTENCIES OF THE INSULIN RESISTANCE THEORY

MEDICAL SCIENTISTS have long been unable to explain many inconsistencies and illogical conclusions about Type 2 diabetes when they use the insulin resistance theory as its cause. My alternative explanation, the "fatty acid burn theory," resolves many of these inconsistencies. Consider the following:

1. *Why don't all obese people develop diabetes?*
   Why doesn't every obese person develop Type 2 diabetes if being overweight is purportedly a causative factor in insulin resistance? The fact that only some obese people develop Type 2 diabetes suggests that some other scientific explanation is needed. The fatty acid burn theory accounts for the answer.

I said earlier that your genes play a big role in your body's ability to store fat, and thus in determining when you might become prediabetic or diabetic. Some people inherit fat cells with a larger capacity for storing fat. These cells take longer to become filled with fat. Other people may have lots of stem cells that can convert to full grown fat cells on demand. The ability of these fat cells to absorb great amounts of fatty acids explains why even some very obese individuals can maintain normal blood glucose levels. Their fat cells can store more fat and their body continues burning glucose for fuel rather than switching to fatty acids, so they do not end up with high blood sugar and diabetes.

2. *Why do thin or lean people get Type 2 diabetes?*

We may equally wonder why lean people can develop Type 2 diabetes, because insulin resistance is often correlated with being triggered when people are overweight. So why would someone who has only a little body fat become a Type 2 diabetic?

The answer is that some people may be born with small capacity fat cells. In comparison to a person with a large body structure and many fat cells, a lean person's fat cells can fill up quickly, initiating the fatty acid burn switch that causes their muscle cells to avoid glucose in favor of burning the fatty acids freely flowing in their bloodstream. And people who have lean ancestors may have inherited fewer fat stem cells. As they gain weight, the rate of conversion of stem cells to fat cells may not occur quickly enough to keep up with the amount of fat being formed.

It is also possible that some people did not receive adequate nutrition in the womb due to a limited intake of food by the mother during pregnancy. As a result, they have a negligible number of cells that were programmed to become fat stem cells. This may predispose them to develop diabetes when they have access to an abundance of food, even when weight charts consider the person to be lean.

3. Why do some women develop diabetes during pregnancy?

Diabetes during pregnancy, called gestational diabetes, has long perplexed medical scientists as it often occurs in women who have no history of diabetes, no family history of diabetes, and no weight problems or other risk factors. These women suddenly develop diabetes during their pregnancy, usually after only 10 to 12 weeks of gestation. But soon after delivery of their baby, often within days, their blood sugar returns to normal. How can this be?

Specialists in hormonal diseases often tell obstetricians that "temporary" insulin resistance causes gestational diabetes. Without proof, obstetricians are supposed to believe that the placenta releases pregnancy hormones and agents that cause insulin resistance in the same three types of cells as regular Type 2 diabetes — fat cells, muscle fibers, and liver cells. This means gestational diabetes is effectively the same as Type 2 diabetes, but it occurs and disappears in a short time.

Using the insulin resistance theory to explain gestational diabetes requires an enormous biological leap of faith: that billions of cells in the body can very quickly develop insulin resistance ... and then just as quickly flip-flop and no longer be insulin resistant. This seems highly implausible and unlikely. And if it is true, why don't the majority of pregnant women develop it?

A better, more logical explanation for gestational diabetes is that in some women, depending on their body build and ancestry, the accumulation of fat from eating occurs faster than the woman's fat cells can accommodate. This leads to the fatty acid burn switch, leaving glucose in the bloodstream. Once the woman delivers, and stops eating as much, she loses weight, fatty acids are stored in fat cells, and her body reverts to burning glucose. This makes far more sense than the insulin resistance theory, given that most (though not all) pregnant women consume food in excess of their normal intake and may temporarily fill up their genetically determined number of fat cells.

In addition, there could be a hormonal trigger here. The hormone cortisol is released during pregnancy, which promotes the release of fatty acids from the fat cells, as well as enhancing fatty acid utilization and stimulating glucose production in the liver. The result is, of course, high levels of sugar in the blood. This explanation for gestational diabetes helps explain why it appears to occur randomly, often in women who have never had high blood sugar or a history of diabetes.

4. *Why are some children younger than 18 developing Type 2 diabetes?*

Without any supporting evidence but pointing only to the symptoms of high levels of glucose and insulin in the blood, it is often stated that some children younger than 18 are now developing insulin resistance leading to Type 2 diabetes. There is no explanation why insulin resistance would develop at such a young age or why the three organs involved are the same as in adult-onset Type 2 diabetes.

The increasing incidence of Type 2 diabetes seen in youth under age 18 can be far better understood with my fatty acid burn theory. In our childhood and teenage years, the body is trying to expand its fat cell supply. Stem cells are being instructed to become fat cells. Many children become obese between the ages of 9 and 15. If the demand for increased storage is not met in a timely fashion, excess fat and fatty acids will stay in the bloodstream. Muscles will start burning fatty acids for energy, while excess amounts of glucose will elevate blood sugar, leading to the development of Type 2 diabetes in children and teens.

5. *Why do statin medicines that lower cholesterol tend to cause diabetes?*

Statins are a class of medication often used to lower cholesterol. Statin use has been associated with an increased risk of Type 2 diabetes, especially in postmenopausal women, as reported after analysis of results among women participating in the Women's Health Initiative.[4] But how are the two metabolisms — cholesterol and glucose — connected? The fatty acid burn theory explains the connection.

First, statins produce their effect by inhibiting the manufacture of cholesterol molecules from fatty acids in the liver. This means that fatty acids which otherwise would have been used for cholesterol formation must be dealt with by the body in other ways. One way is that the liver uses these fatty acids to produce triglycerides, which are transported to fat cells where they are stored. This is not a problem for people whose fat cells have the storage capacity.

However, for people whose fat cells are already filled, they end up with excess fatty acids from the triglycerides that have nowhere to go. And of course, this then triggers the fatty acid burn switch, when muscles change to burn fatty acids for fuel rather than glucose, creating high blood sugar and Type 2 diabetes.

6. *How exactly do our genes cause Type 2 diabetes?*

It is believed that diabetes is genetic because insulin resistance is passed from one generation to the next. But again, there is no proof of this. The supposed mechanism that links genetic obesity and insulin resistance in cells has not been identified. No defective genes have been found that link the two together. In addition, there is no explanation for why thin individuals develop Type 2 diabetes. If they are not obese, why would they develop insulin resistance since they experienced no weight gain? And if the explanation has something to do with being thin, why didn't they develop insulin resistance at a younger age?

My fatty acid burn theory provides a far better explanation for why diabetes is genetic. It has nothing to do with insulin resistance, but rather with how your genetic inheritance dictates your ability to store fat and how quickly your fat cells fill up. Your genes may have given you large fat cells that fill up slowly, thus avoiding or delaying diabetes forever or at least for decades. Or your genes may have endowed you with very few fat cells, so they fill up quickly, causing your muscles to switch to burning fatty acids from your bloodstream rather than glucose. Your genes thus dictate, without your knowing, if and when you might develop high blood sugar.

The Role of Genes in Type 2 Diabetes

A gene can be defined as a packet of instructions to manufacture functional products needed inside a cell in the body. This view of the role of genes helps us better understand who gets diabetes and who doesn't in a family. Although all humans have similar genes, genes that are active within each cell are different from person to person.

Consider two siblings in a family where one parent is heavyset and diabetic and the other lean and non-diabetic. Each parent contributes one-half of each pair of genes in every cell in the offspring's body. Which gene of each pair becomes active depends on many factors during the development of the fetus.

In one sibling, for instance, genes inherited from the heavyset parent could produce more fat cells and/or larger fat cells that can store more fat. This sibling could have a greater capacity to store fat and become heavier than the other sibling. The glucose and fatty acid levels in the blood could appear normal because they are stored in the fat cells. This sibling might never develop Type 2 diabetes.

The other sibling, however, despite being considered lean based on a standardized weight table, could develop Type 2 diabetes because they have genes that produced limited fat storage capacity. This sibling could fill up all their fat cells by the time he or she is 35 or 40, triggering the switch from glucose to fatty acid burn in muscle cells.

From this perspective, we might logically conclude that inherited genes do play a role in determining who develops Type 2 diabetes. But the difference between my theory and the standard theory of diabetes is that genetics does not cause insulin resistance to occur. Type 2 diabetes is a function of the body's genetically determined capability to store fat. How fast and how early in life one's potential fat storage capacity is used up varies by individual.

Another factor of genetics that could play a role as a direct cause of diabetes is our attitude and behaviors around eating. We know that our genes play a role in determining our ability to cope with stress and emotional difficulties. People who become diabetic may have a genetic predisposition to become easily stressed out. Through genetics and family upbringing, they may deal with stress by eating, even when not hungry. Our reactions to stress and our eating habits are often a function of our personality, which is influenced by our genes. We will be discussing the issue of stress and changing your eating behaviors later in the book.

Yet another factor to consider is the effect of environment on activation of gene(s). An example of this interaction between the environment and genes is the increasing incidence of Type 2 diabetes in countries like India and China where for generations people have been of shorter stature, on an average, compared to those in the West, possibly because of limited availability of food. This means potentially lower fat storage capacity. Meanwhile, the recent increased availability and affordability of food in general, and grain-based foods in particular, makes it possible for more and more people to fill their fat stores at a younger and younger age, leading to the development of diabetes. It may take a few generations of overeating before the genetic capability of increased fat storage can be widespread in these countries.

Keep in mind that genes only confer the potential for something to happen, similar to the capability of an engine in a car to go at various speeds. At what speed the car travels is up to the driver to decide. In other words, how fast one fills up the fat storage capacity is a function of each individual and the environment in which he or she lives. Thus, even if diabetes appears in various members within a family, it need not be based on genetic inheritance but on factors such as eating grain-based foods multiple times daily.

Why does Type 2 diabetes sometimes disappear after weight loss?

My alternate explanation makes far more sense than crediting the sudden disappearance of insulin resistance to weight loss. When you lose weight, it's evident that your fat cells get rid of their stores of triglycerides. The empty fat cells can now accept new triglycerides made by the liver from glucose and fatty acids absorbed after a meal. Muscles can revert to using glucose more often for energy because fewer fatty acids are circulating in the blood since they are being stored inside fat cells. Blood sugar can be maintained within a normal range.

WHY DO DIABETES MEDICATIONS SEEM TO WORK IF INSULIN RESISTANCE IS NOT THE CAUSE?

THE PRIMARY objective of any medical management program is to cure an ailment. To achieve a cure, one needs to know the cause. However, when it comes to Type 2 diabetes, the cause and mechanism of insulin resistance are unknown.

For this reason, drug companies have had to take many approaches to develop medications to "control" blood sugar. Pharmaceutical companies perform years of tests, but government approval of medications for sale does not mean that chemists and scientists truly understand how a specific drug impacts an organ. For example, in the case of insulin resistance in cells, there is still no specific test that proves how that resistance happens and how medications are supposedly correcting it.

Furthermore, the word "control" used for diabetes only means keeping blood sugar closer to the normal range. In my view, controlling blood sugar through medications is of questionable value, as it under-mines the assessment of long-term diabetes management.[5] Take fever, the common marker of an infection in the body, for example. We can determine the effectiveness of a medication such as aspirin or acetamin-ophen by measuring changes in a patient's fever. A person who took aspi-rin to lower a 102-degree fever to just 99 degrees is doing better, but it does not necessarily mean that the infection is under control. The med-ication treated only the symptoms, but not the cause of the infection.

For the same reason, many diabetes medications may lower blood sugar, but they do not do anything to treat the supposed insulin resis-tance. The lack of precise knowledge about what insulin resistance is explains why no diabetes medication has ever been able to reverse the unproven cause of insulin resistance.

The illogic of some medications

There is also a highly illogical explanation for certain medications. Think of it this way: as a rule, if a person with a bacterial infection becomes resistant to an antibiotic, the doctor must switch and use a different antibiotic to treat the condition. Similarly, if a cancer patient becomes resistant to a chemotherapy agent, the doctor changes the medication. Yet, diabetes experts continue to prescribe medications that cause the release of more insulin from one's own pancreas or pre-scribe injections of insulin into the body in an attempt to "overcome" insulin resistance in a patient with Type 2 diabetes.

So ask yourself: if cells are resistant to insulin, why flood them with more of it? Isn't that illogical? How can they be sensitive to more insulin if they are insulin resistant?

The fact that some medications reduce blood sugar does not spe-cifically support the insulin resistance theory. When a patient takes such a medication and experiences lower blood sugar, there is no guar-antee that glucose molecules have gotten inside the cells that had been resistant to insulin. Without evidence, diabetes experts claim that the sugar was metabolized, but they are not truly clarifying how the glucose was utilized or which cells absorbed the glucose molecules. In fact, it's possible that other body cells that were sensitive to insulin all along may have absorbed more glucose. If so, how does that help the patient?

Finally, there is a serious danger with medications that put the pancreas on overdrive. Like every organ, the pancreas has a finite operational working capacity and life. Although it can last for an entire human lifetime, forcing it to work at a greater volume than normal can cause more harm than good. It could lead to an early exhaustion of the pancreatic cells that produce and secrete insulin. In addition, allowing patients to adjust the dose of their medications often encourages them to continue the same lifestyle of eating the wrong foods and overeating grains, thinking their diabetes is "under control" when, in fact, they are only shifting glucose out of the blood circulation but not out of the body. When glucose remains in the body, it triggers the complications of diabetes.

In short, in Type 2 diabetes, the cells are never resistant to insulin; cells did not need glucose at that time, but medications force them to take glucose in.

Other types of diabetes medications

Several other diabetes medications function in a different way to lower blood sugar, although again, none of them resolve the cause of the supposed insulin resistance.

Medications that increase insulin sensitivity — Some diabetic medications are supposed to facilitate the entry of glucose into cells in the body by increasing their "insulin sensitivity," or, phrased another way, by decreasing the "insulin resistance" of the organs. However, even the pharmaceutical companies that make these drugs have not identified the mechanisms by which this feat is accomplished.

In my view, there are serious questions about medications that increase insulin sensitivity. Is it a good thing to increase insulin sensitivity in the three types of cells responsible for diabetes — muscle, liver, and fat cells? If muscle cells become more insulin sensitive, will they be able to absorb more glucose? And if a person does not exercise to burn that glucose, what happens to all the glucose in the muscle cells? If the liver becomes more insulin sensitive, it should produce more triglycerides using glucose, but where will those triglycerides be stored? And is it beneficial to transform glucose, which is water-soluble and can leave the body in the urine, into triglycerides that are not water-soluble and can stick to arterial walls and potentially obstruct the person's flow of blood? If fat cells become more insulin sensitive, will they just store more fat? Can they store an unlimited amount?

Medications that create new fat cells to store excess glucose — One class of medications lowers blood sugar by inducing faster formation of new fat cells to create a larger storage area. These drugs do not affect the insulin resistance theory since they have nothing to do with altering insulin production or improving insulin sensitivity. In fact, this drug approach to treating diabetes supports my fatty acid burn theory because the drugs work by increasing storage for fatty acids, allowing cells to switch back to burning glucose.

But such medications have proved to work only temporarily, because eventually the patient's newly formed fat cells also fill to capacity, especially if the person continues to overconsume grains. Once this happens, it has proved that these medications stop being effective in lowering blood sugar levels.

Medications that prevent the digestion of carbohydrates in the intestine, or prevent the release of glucose from the liver, or that speed up elimination of glucose through the urine — These drugs do not negate the fatty acid burn theory, nor do they support the insulin resistance theory. These types of medications have many troubling side effects, such as indigestion or increasing the excretion of water through the kidney, which can lead to dehydration. It would be healthier for a prediabetic or diabetic to eat less carbohydrate and produce less glucose than to risk those side effects.

Insulin injections

Doctors usually treat people who have been diagnosed as fully diabetic over a long period of time and whose blood sugar levels remain very high by having them take insulin injections. In some instances, such patients already have low levels of natural insulin from years of taking other medications that have exhausted the ability of their pancreas to produce insulin. In some countries, doctors immediately prescribe insulin injections, even if patients were only recently diagnosed, perhaps because of the convenience of administering a precise dosage to achieve a desired blood sugar level. In addition, patients feel empowered to be able to decide the insulin dose based on the amount of carbohydrate consumed during a meal.

For most people with diabetes, especially those with a busy lifestyle, measured doses of insulin put directly into the body using a device or a pump is far more convenient and easier than making changes in their eating habits. Pharmaceutical companies encourage this attitude by marketing insulin preparations that are long-lasting, such that only one injection per day is needed. What is missing from this line of thinking, in my opinion, is the awareness of other biological activities of insulin that can lead to undesired results.

As explained earlier, one of these is the role that insulin plays in causing cancer to occur in cells. It is established that as the prevalence of Type 2 diabetes is increasing worldwide, so is that of cancer. Epidemiological studies show that liver and pancreatic cancers have a strong relationship with diabetes, perhaps because both organs play a central role in blood sugar regulation, which makes them susceptible to the presence of insulin, which, whether released internally or injected into the body, acts as a growth promoter for cells. The problem is, insulin can also accelerate the multiplication of cancer cells that appear at random in the body of a person with diabetes. Effectively, the more insulin you put into your body, the more risk you take to create the conditions for cancer cell growth. Meanwhile, high levels of circulating glucose also contribute to this because cancer cells use glucose as their primary fuel to produce energy for their growth, multiplication, and migration to other sites in the body.

Why it's better to avoid diabetes medications

If you are not yet taking medication for high blood sugar, your best option is to read the rest of this book and begin implementing the 8 steps that I will be teaching you. This begins by changing your eating habits to severely limit grains and grain-flour products. This is the first key to getting and remaining off diabetic medications.

Believe me, it is vital that you avoid diabetes medications because taking them can lead to the formation of more fat — and eventually to weight gain — because medicine-induced higher insulin production causes the liver to convert more glucose to triglycerides in the effort to keep your blood sugar in check. So, in effect, taking medication harms you more than it solves anything.

If you are already taking a medication that supposedly helps you with insulin resistance, you too will want to work towards stopping it by implementing the advice in this book. By altering your diet to minimize grain-based foods, you will be able to lower your blood sugar and work with your doctor to reduce to zero your use of diabetic medications.

The reason I suggest you avoid medications to control blood sugar is, again, that they simply target the wrong problem. No medication has been shown to stop your body from becoming insulin resistant, which in my view is proof that science has yet to identify the mechanism by which this resistance occurs, which should put doubt in our minds that it even exists.

In addition, many medications create undesirable immediate side effects, even at low dosage levels. Doctors often prescribe other medications to deal with those side effects, so you end up on a slippery slope to needing more and more medications.

Finally, the use of medications to overcome high blood sugar does not guarantee that diabetic complications won't develop. Many diabetic patients spend decades taking medications or injecting insulin, yet they succumb to atherosclerosis, which leads to heart attack, stroke, and amputation of limbs; diabetic neuropathy; loss of eyesight; kidney failure and the need for dialysis; impotence in men; and diabetic coma.

The politics of making Type 2 diabetes a disease

The usual method of validating any scientific theory is through logic, mechanism, and measurement to establish proof of concept. Unfortunately, even after 80 years of acceptance of insulin resistance, no one knows the logic behind why only 3 types of cells out of more than 200 types become resistant to insulin, or the mechanism of that resistance in relation to metabolic activities that differ in each site. Nor do we have a test to measure the degree of resistance at any one of the sites.

Yet, the concept of insulin resistance has spawned an enormous number of research papers, one after another that simply rely on preceding papers to establish their credibility. The sheer volume of these papers has forced acceptance by the medical community at large, who then put it forth as a validated theory for the general public.

Many of the research papers were made possible by funding from companies with vested interest, especially pharmaceutical companies that are willing to keep the insulin resistance theory alive because they are profiting enormously selling drugs that are supposed to improve insulin sensitivity or force release of pancreatic insulin; supplying patients with insulin injections of different strengths and durations of action; and making methods of insulin administration more convenient. This creates the illusion that the patient is in fact controlling his or her condition just by keeping blood sugar levels within acceptable limits.

These companies make billions of dollars on their medications and are not inclined to fund research that challenges the insulin resistance theory. Other companies benefit from the production and sale of meters and test strips for measuring blood glucose at home. Diabetes has also spawned many powerful, well-funded organizations that promulgate the insulin resistance explanation about diabetes — and only this one. They organize meetings, produce leaflets, distribute magazines, help publish books, create audiovisual materials, publish treatment guidelines, provide certified educators to make patients understand the complexity of their condition and accept the permanency of it, and instruct family members and friends to make sure that patients accept this single explanation. These organizations serve the public in many ways but are they doing so responsibly if they are not considering other explanations or questioning treatment objectives based primarily on improvements in a patient's laboratory values? Over time, such organizations become more interested in protecting their turf than striving for better patient outcomes.

I am reluctant to discuss the politics of diabetes in such a cynical way, but we must begin recognizing that big corporations are influencing our healthcare decisions because they want to preserve their profits. The claim of insulin resistance and the management of Type 2 diabetes based on that concept will persist for the foreseeable future unless it is exposed as unscientific.

Medical management through fear

The real tragedy of using medications to control Type 2 diabetes is that it engenders fear. Patients are usually given the scary news that they have an "irreversible and incurable" condition called insulin resistance, and that Type 2 diabetes is a "progressive disease." The message is presented as if it is clearly understood by experts who, in reality, cannot prove it scientifically.

Some people with severe diabetes also fear its corollary problem, hypoglycemia — when blood sugar goes too low, causing many serious symptoms. This fear often compels them to eat even when they are not hungry, or to eat more than they need to because their medical caregiver told them to do so.

Many medical practitioners use fear to encourage diabetic patients to check their blood glucose level daily at home. Their idea is that the more accurately you know your blood sugar level, the better you can control it. However, there are no studies showing that regularly checking your blood sugar level results in better long-term maintenance of the blood sugar levels, a lower incidence of hypoglycemia, or fewer complications of Type 2 diabetes.

I am opposed to most medications to control blood sugar in prediabetics and in people in the early stage of Type 2 diabetes with no other complications. My view is that medical treatment for Type 2 diabetes should be based on achieving the most significant beneficial outcomes. These include the reduced risk of having problems related to the heart, eye, kidney, and other organs — not any supposed evidence that your blood sugar values have declined. Many people taking diabetes medications to lower blood sugar still end up with lost eyesight, amputations, kidney disease, or other serious complications.

In the end, this means that, if you are seeking a reversal of diabetes, it is important to greatly reduce or even eliminate grains and grain-flour products from your diet. This action cuts down the excess glucose that your body has to store in the form of triglyceride. Once your fat cells are full, the body is programmed to burn fatty acids instead of glucose to produce energy, leaving glucose in the blood leading to Type 2 diabetes. Minimizing your consumption of grains and grain-flour products, on the other hand, reduces the accumulation of fatty acids flowing in the bloodstream, so your body can revert to the normal pattern of burning glucose in your muscle cells. You will thus put an end to the fatty acid burn switch, lowering the level of glucose in your blood.

A warning for those taking insulin injections

For Type 1 diabetics, insulin is a lifesaver.

In people with Type 1 diabetes, the objective of insulin administration is very clear and the benefits such as improved quality of life and prolonged lifespan are fully understood and documented.

For Type 2 diabetics, insulin is a troublemaker.

• Insulin causes you to be hungry.

When blood glucose level is lowered as a result of insulin administration, one of the symptoms experienced is the sensation of hunger. If you are asked to lose weight as part of your treatment strategy for diabetes, how can the administration of an agent that makes you hungry be helpful?

• Mistakes in using insulin can be deadly.

There are many practical difficulties in determining the dose and timing of insulin administration for precise control of blood sugar. For example, insulin preparations differ in durations of action, and the amount of carbohydrates one unit of insulin can handle varies almost threefold between different people. It is impossible to match the body's natural rhythmic release mechanism of insulin by any methodology currently available for insulin administration.

For example, if the body senses a sharp drop in blood sugar level because of insulin, it causes the release of another pancreatic hormone, glucagon, which instructs the liver to release glucose into the blood. The presence of stress and illness is another confounder in determining the correct dose. The variability of absorption of insulin into the bloodstream from the site of injection is yet another factor.

Thus, if your insulin dose administered turns out to be incorrect, or if you fail to consume the expected amount of food after taking the normal dosage, you could experience severe hypoglycemia. If this happens when you are under the influence of alcohol or sleeping medication, vital control centers in the brain may stop functioning due to lack of glucose availability. You may never wake up from sleep.

• Taking insulin for insulin resistance is illogical.

It is a common medical practice not to administer an antibiotic if a person with an infection is found to be resistant to it. It is also common to withhold a chemotherapeutic agent from a patient resistant to it. However, when it comes to Type 2 diabetes, endocrinologists advocate administering insulin to a person supposedly resistant to insulin, in an attempt to "overcome" the resistance. How this is accomplished has never been clarified. In addition, there aren't any tests to measure the degree of insulin resistance at any of the affected sites, before and after insulin administration.

• Taking insulin does not guarantee against the consequences of diabetes.

Even when you diligently adjust your insulin dose and keep your blood sugar within the desired levels, there is no guarantee that you will not suffer the same types of complications of Type 2 diabetes people with poorly controlled blood sugar. Statistics do not show that insulin injections prevent people from damage to nerve cells, blindness, kidney failure, atherosclerosis, and diabetic coma.

• Insulin promotes cancer.

Insulin is a known promoter of cell growth including the growth of cancer cells. The presence of insulin either injected into the body or released in response to another agent administered can promote the growth of cancer cells in the body.

• Taking insulin leads you to believe you are in control (but you're not). Diabetes experts and drug companies equate and advertise controlling blood sugar as successful diabetes treatment. But this profit-oriented advertising often incentivizes diabetics to believe they do not need to make dietary changes to lose weight or lower blood sugar by avoiding the consumption of grains. You may also like the convenience of long-acting injections and give in to thinking you can control your diabetes, but you are still at risk for diabetes consequences and cancer.

Caution: If you decide to follow the recommendations in this book to significantly reduce grains and grain-based carbohydrates from your diet, please be sure to reduce the dose of your insulin, especially the evening dose, to avoid blood sugar levels becoming too low during your sleep. For more information on how to change your medications as you alter your diet, see Appendix 3.

THE REAL CURE

8 STEPS TO REVERSE
TYPE 2 DIABETES
IN 8 WEEKS

REDUCE GRAINS CONSIDERABLY FROM YOUR DIET

YOU HAVE learned that insulin resistance is not the cause of high blood sugar and diabetes, so let's turn our attention to how you can reverse these conditions. You know that the real culprit in causing high blood sugar is the consumption of grains and grain-flour products. Those foods are usually in your diet, often for every meal. It starts with the cereal, toast, muffin, sweet roll, or oatmeal you eat at breakfast, then the sandwich you eat for lunch, then a heavy dinner almost always with a heaping serving of rice or corn, plus perhaps a sauce that contains flour, and a dinner roll on the side, and then topped off with cake or pie.

If this or something similar sounds like your usual diet, you are consuming an excessive amount of grain-based carbohydrate that converts to more glucose than your body can immediately use or store. Added to many people's food choices are the pizzas, doughnuts, cookies, and other foods made with flour that are consumed regularly. It is therefore no wonder that diabetes is spreading at pandemic levels in the US as well as in many nations of the world.

As the figure below shows, grains break down into hundreds of thousands of molecules of glucose.

STARCH/FLOUR

Starch is made from glucose molecules linked to each other in complex ways. Each molecule of flour (starch) you eat may contain up to 200,000 glucose molecules, tightly packed.

Let me boil the science down for you to the key recommendation in changing your diet to reverse your diabetes:

> *Lower your consumption of grains as much as you can.*
> *Cut grains down to less than 20% of your daily caloric intake.*

Considerably reduce your consumption of wheat, oats, rye, corn, rice, and other grains. Don't be persuaded by secondary advertising claims such as "no cholesterol," "gluten free," "fortified with vitamins and minerals," "whole grain" or "multigrain" and "no high-fructose corn syrup" because such claims do not change the basic result of digesting these products — they are still foods that will elevate your blood sugar.

When I tell people this, their first reaction is usually focused on some fear they have about giving up eating these. "I'm going to be hungry if I don't eat bread, pasta, or rice." There are those who exclaim: "I won't have any energy without bread and other carbs." Another common reaction is: "How can I possibly live without the convenience of bread to make sandwiches?" These are things you might be saying to yourself right now, worried you will be entering a new life without grain-based foods that is almost unimaginable to you.

These fears make people reluctant to change. But if you are willing to listen, learn, and consider a change in your lifestyle, you can truly lower your blood sugar and reverse your diabetes. You will probably also lose weight, feel healthier, and have more energy. So why not give it a try?

From this point on, start decreasing your consumption of grains. Cut them out of your diet day-by-day, moving as close to zero consumption as possible. While consuming small amounts of grain and grain-flour products once in a while, such as a small bowl of oatmeal or a slice of bread, every few days is acceptable, it is best to move towards significantly reducing how much you eat of grain-based cereals, granolas, muffins, croissants, sweet pastries, sandwiches, and other grain-flour items of food each and every day. Instead, use food preparations made from fresh vegetables, fruit, nuts, eggs, dairy, and meat. For lunches, cut out on several days per week sandwiches on breads (see sidebar, *Living Without Sandwiches*). Choose instead salads, lettuce wraps, or wraps made with non-grain products. Order a fresh fish plate with vegetables, a burger wrapped in lettuce without a bun, or vegetables and a dip like hummus. At dinner, stop serving rice, corn, wheat-based pastas, and dinner rolls. In place of those, cook up lentils or beans, adding spices to flavor them to match your main dish, plus a fresh vegetable or a mixed salad.

There are thousands of recipes available for side dishes made with legumes such as lentils and beans as well as recipes for cooked vegetables and fresh salads.

In short, it's entirely possible to transform your diet to reduce grains and grain-based foods and still enjoy cooking and eating many types of foods. To help you in this endeavor, I have published the *Diabetes-Free Cookbook & Exercise Guide* that contains over 80 delicious recipes and 12 easy-to-do exercises. The recipes in this book were created by a professional chef working with me to develop delicious breakfasts, lunches, dinners, and snacks that are almost entirely grain-free.

The fear of feeling hungry without grains

Feeling hungry can be more intense than many other human feelings or desires. It drives us to form behavior patterns that often lead to eating foods that make us feel happy by overeating until we are uncomfortably full. The reason that grain products give you the sensation of fullness is that they absorb water and swell up in your stomach, not because they provide nutrition to stop your hunger. Many people need to experience a bloated stomach to feel they had a satisfying meal. Some people will counterargue that for hundreds of years, people have consumed rice and flat breads made with rice, wheat, or corn flour without having high blood sugar or diabetes. So what changed? Let me explain.

Tens of thousands of years ago, humans consumed flat bread made with starch extracted from the roots of plants. Cultivation of rice and wheat began only about 10,000 years ago. Only in the past 100 years has increased production of grains become possible with the use of better seeds, synthetic fertilizers, pesticides, mechanized farming, efficient water management, and government subsidies to farmers. Modern milling and refining methods resulted in grain flours with varied physical characteristics making it possible for chefs and homemakers to create a multitude of breads and other dishes.

REDUCE GRAINS CONSIDERABLY FROM YOUR DIET

Therefore, it is not surprising that bread prepared from dough made with flour and water is one of the most common foods eaten with almost every meal, or as a snack, or used as an ingredient in other food preparations. Food assistance programs have made it easier for nearly everyone on earth, even in developing countries, to have access to grains and grain-flour products. In addition, many people are misled by believing that if they eat "whole grain" or "multigrain" products, they are eating healthy. The fact is, although whole grains and grain-flour products may contain bran with B vitamins, they are mostly made of molecules of glucose.

Over the past few decades, the quantity of grain and grain-flour foods consumed by most individuals is far more than what can be utilized for energy between meals or stored in fat cells in the body.

The cure is to severely reduce grains. You *can* eat a meal with practically no bread, corn, rice, or other grains. My suggestion is to go back to how people were eating about 100 years ago, before cultivated grains became a staple of the common diet. For example, before large-scale grain farming started, humans met their energy and nutrient needs from fruits, roots, nuts, peas, lentils, chickpeas, vegetables, dairy products, eggs, fish and other items from the sea, mushrooms, and small and large animal meats, without much reliance on grain-based products such as we consume today.

Can you live without sandwiches?

If you take this advice, you will quickly learn that, yes, life can go on without sandwiches. If you avoid most grains that are used as sandwich holders or wrappers, you will decrease your chances of developing high blood sugar and eventually becoming diabetic.

I acknowledge that you may find this difficult to do at first. You might have grown up eating sandwiches of all kinds, and you enjoy them as a frequent part of your diet. Sandwiches are convenient ways to combine meats, vegetables, and condiments into a tasty package. They are affordable and easy to make or purchase, to carry with you, and to eat at your desk, in the car, or on the go. They make lunchtime with colleagues in the park or in a little sandwich shop the simplest way to eat and chat. I know very well how any type of food item can become so ingrained in your mind that it appears unimaginable to give it up.

But let me ask you to be honest with yourself: would you rather continue consuming sandwiches made with grain-based breads for convenience and end up having diabetes for life? Or would you rather look at creative ways you can enjoy food without the need for sandwich bread so you can reverse your diabetes and feel healthy?

I very much hope you will opt for the latter choice. A life of high blood sugar, medications, and the worsening complications of diabetes over decades as you age is just not worth the convenience of eating sandwiches.

There are many natural products that can be used as the "holder" or "platform" for vegetables and meat. People of many different cultures have long used lettuce, cabbage, and even grape leaves to hold food. Breads and crackers made with lentil or garbanzo bean flour are now available. Although these legumes contain carbohydrates, these escape from digestion in the small intestine of healthy individuals while providing the benefits of adding fiber to your diet. Many fast-food outlets today let you purchase their foods wrapped in lettuce, with no bun. Pizza crusts and bread made from cauliflower or other vegetables with absolutely no wheat or other grain-flour ingredients are another option to use in place of bread. You can also transform your normal sandwich ingredients into a salad.

Start today: go sandwich-free for just a week. If you are afraid of experiencing "sandwich withdrawal," you will find that within a short time, you will not crave eating as many sandwiches as you formerly consumed. You will look in the mirror and see yourself shedding pounds and feeling healthier and more energetic. And, best of all, you will see your blood sugar level drop as you begin to reverse your diabetes.

The fear of feeling tired by not eating grains

Many people are concerned that they may not have the energy necessary for their daily tasks if they don't eat to fullness during a meal. The first thing to remember is that each pound of fat stored in your body represents 3500 calories, far more than you would ordinarily spend in a day. In other words, your body's energy needs are generally fulfilled with very little food, far less than you probably consume each day.

Unless you are an athlete working out all day long, or your job is very physically demanding and burns a lot of energy in a short period of time, you can survive and thrive on just two or three modest meals per day or, if you prefer, multiple smaller meals. You do not need to consume grain-based foods to feel energetic.

Consumption of grains and grain-based foods makes most people gain weight by adding pounds of fat made from the unused glucose that must be stored in your fat cells. The permanent extra weight, usually added at a rate of one or two pounds a year, is what makes you feel tired. In addition, the overconsumption of grains and grain-based foods makes you feel tired immediately after a meal when the body responds by releasing a robust amount of insulin to clear the blood of excess glucose.

Take breakfast, for example, considered by some as the most important meal of the day. How much carbohydrate do you need to eat at breakfast to recharge your energy after sleeping, without undue elevation of blood sugar and insulin? Since the liver can store only 120 grams of glucose as glycogen (the storage form of complex carbohydrate to be released into the blood when blood sugar level dips), the amount of carbohydrate needs to match only what has been depleted in the night (or whatever time of the day) when you slept.

A rough estimate can be made if one assumes a steady release of glucose from the liver on an hourly basis. Since 120 grams of glucose represents 30 teaspoons of sugar (there are 4 grams of sugar per teaspoon), fasting overnight for 12 hours will require only one half of the liver's capacity — 15 teaspoons of complex carbohydrate — to replenish its stores.

This is only an estimate, but your brain knows the actual need and will help you to better quantity control, based on how you eat. For example, if you slowly eat a fresh fruit, your brain knows the amount of carbohydrate consumed based on the registration of fruit sugar by your sweet-tasting taste buds. You may also eat some meat or eggs, if desired, to provide the body with other needed nutrients.

You will see that even when reducing grain and grain-flour products, you will have enough energy to do your daily activities without feeling tired while keeping your blood sugar level within normal limits.

Is eating any grains OK?

Often people who do not want to give up grain-based foods but are willing to change their eating habit ask what type of grain is better for them to consume. This is similar to the question asked by an alcohol addict whether alcohol from beer is better than that from wine or distilled spirits. As you can imagine, the chemical nature of alcohol is the same whether you consume it in any of the three forms mentioned. However, the percentage can vary from 5% in beer, 10–15% in wine, and 40–55% in spirits.

Glucose molecules are similar, regardless of the grain they come from. However, per 100–gram portion (about 7 tablespoons), the carbohydrate content can vary from 80% in white rice to 71% in wheat. Some foods that people consume because they are not considered true grains are almost as high in carbohydrate content per 100 grams, such as buckwheat (71%) and quinoa (64%), although this makes them slightly healthier for you.

So, the real question is how much are you going to eat? As you can see, 100 grams of rice, wheat, or even quinoa provides a significant amount of carbohydrate that will be absorbed as glucose into the body. If you remember simply that 4 grams = 1 teaspoon of sugar (glucose), consider these examples:

- 100 grams of rice at 80% carbohydrate = 80 grams of carbohydrate = 20 teaspoons of sugar
- 100 grams of quinoa at 64% carbohydrate = 64 grams of carbohydrate = 16 teaspoons of sugar

Calculating your intake can become very confusing if you try to account for the actual percentage of carbohydrate in a serving of grains or pseudo-grains like quinoa and buckwheat. It is far simpler and healthier to err on the safe side and just remember this basic ratio which I have rounded off for simplicity:

4 grams of any grain = 1 teaspoon of sugar = 4 grams of stored glucose

Given that liver only holds 120 grams of glucose stored as glycogen at a time, any meal that includes more than about 120 grams of carbohydrate intake will produce excess glucose your body cannot utilize immediately and will need to be stored as fat. (This assumes that the liver has exhausted all its glycogen reserves, which is usually not the case.) If not utilized at some time, this excess glucose will eventually fill your fat cells and cause the switch to burning fatty acids, leaving you with high blood sugar and diabetes.

See Appendix 1 for more information on how grains compare to fruits and vegetables as the source of carbohydrates. This will help you understand why eating fresh vegetables and fruit, along with fish, meat, and dairy as you wish, is a better choice to help lower your blood sugar and reverse your diabetes.

RECONNECT WITH YOUR AUTHENTIC WEIGHT

THE NEXT 7 STEPS are aimed at how you can begin to make other necessary changes to your diet and eating habits to normalize your blood sugar, reverse your diabetes, and maintain these behavioral changes for good health and a long life.

Reconnecting with your authentic weight

If you want to commit long-term to a new diet and eating habits, it begins with reconnecting with your "authentic" weight. I believe that every person has access to a wise method for determining if you are carrying too much fat in your body, which sets the stage for the switch from glucose to fatty acids as the fuel your muscles burn. This method is what I call "feeling your authentic weight."

Whenever I tell people about this concept, almost everyone knows exactly what I am talking about. It is intuitive and immediate — and I assume you understood it as soon as you read it in the same way that you automatically know what people mean when they talk about "justice" or "equality" or "morality" without their having to define it. We all have a sense of our authentic weight because our brain tells us what it should be.

Perhaps you have never thought about your authentic weight, but once you begin reflecting on it, and being honest with yourself, you will develop a good sense of what it should be. Becoming mindful about your authentic weight connects you to your brain's way of signaling that you are exceeding the weight that is right for you.

When you are in tune with your authentic weight, you immediately sense it when you gain a few extra pounds because you start to feel uncomfortable at first. Your stomach feels distended or bloated, you may feel some muscle pains, or you may feel slower and tired more often.

When you exceed your authentic weight, you will usually find yourself thinking something like, "Gosh, I'm getting heavy. Maybe I need to lose a pound or two."

Unfortunately, most people tend to rationalize away their weight gain once they exceed their authentic weight by a few pounds. They attribute it to stress, aging, busy days at work, family obligations, lack of time to exercise, the discovery of a new food they love to eat, or simply that other people around them are gaining weight, too. They believe they will easily lose weight soon enough and so do not worry about it.

Such rationalization becomes increasingly convincing over time because your brain tends to believe ideas it repeats. In fact, many people even consciously overeat at a meal, believing that the next day, they will compensate for it by eating less. But they don't. Little by little, year by year, they put on pounds, using a continuous loop of overeating, rationalization, and reneging on their commitment to eat less in the coming days and months.

It helps to understand more about body weight to overcome this rationalization. Your authentic body weight is a measure of the total mass of all components of your body including bone, muscle, organs, blood, fat, and water. The role of each of these components in contributing to one's weight differs in every individual in the world. You could be tall and small boned with lots of muscle, or short and big boned with regular muscle — and weigh the same. Only you can intuitively know your authentic weight based on what your brain assesses and tells you (if you are willing to listen).

Your authentic weight can also change as you exercise and age, because the contributions of each component of weight can change. If you begin working out, adding muscle, you might gain muscle weight, but your brain knows you are still in your authentic range because it takes into account your extra muscle mass. If you are aging and losing muscle, but gain 10 pounds in body fat, your brain will sense that your authentic weight is now skewed towards fat, even though you may weigh the same. That is what gives you the sense that you are now uncomfortable with your weight.

Why you cannot use weight charts or the Body Mass Index

You may wonder, why not just use the standard weight tables as a guide to determine your authentic weight?

You are probably not aware that the most common weight guidelines used by doctors in the US are based on data originally obtained in 1943 from the Metropolitan Life Insurance Company (MetLife). The tables were made because MetLife was trying to calculate the insurance risk of people dying. The company asked their policyholders to self-report their height and weight when they purchased life insurance, and they then used that data to prepare a chart of "ideal" weights based on the lowest mortality rates among their customers. People who lived the longest were deemed to have been at the ideal weight when they filled out the survey at the age they were. However, these weight tables are not scientific; there is no definitive linkage between weight and mortality, so these weight tables are effectively useless.

In 1985, a new height and weight chart was prepared by the Gerontology Research Center, National Institute of Aging, Baltimore,

Maryland, which attempted to calculate a healthy weight range for adults of all ages. The problem with this newer chart is that the range of weights for each height is very broad, but it does not significantly help in predicting whether someone might become diabetic. No one has been able to pinpoint a clear "cut-off" point in any weight range that determines what extra amount of weight triggers high blood sugar.

For example, let's say you are 35 years old, stand at 5 feet, 5 inches tall and weigh 145 pounds. The 1985 height/weight chart says you are normal, as you fit inside the bracket between 115 and 149 pounds. But let's say that after developing diabetes, you succeed at losing 12 pounds to weigh just 135 pounds, and your blood sugar returns to normal. How could you have known that your non-diabetic weight should have been at the lower end of the range rather than the higher end?

Body fat ratio and the Body Mass Index (BMI)

Another weight guideline some people use is the ratio of body fat to weight. This can help predict the risk of diabetes in a person because it provides some indication of how much body fat you are carrying. One method used to measure body fat is underwater weighing.

The differences in the densities of fat, muscle, and bone allow an accurate determination of the percentage of body fat. However, this method of measuring your body fat ratio doesn't indicate the location of your fat distribution, i.e., the amount of fat in each location of your body, which helps to understand the potential fullness of your fat cells.

A cheaper and faster measure is the Body Mass Index (BMI), based on a mathematically derived formula that considers the effect of your height on your body weight. More height generally means more bone and muscle that weigh more. So this measure is a little better because statistics show that people who have a greater percentage of bone and muscle tend to have a lower BMI than those with a higher percentage of body fat. You can measure your BMI at the website for the National Heart, Lung, and Blood Institute.[6]

However, the BMI test can be misleading, as its formula cannot distinguish fat mass from muscle mass. Muscles weigh more than fat. This means that if you are very muscular at any height, it adds to your weight, skewing your BMI. A test might indicate that you are overweight or obese, when in fact you are not. The reading would be false if it indicated you are at risk for diabetes just because your BMI is high.

The BMI test can also underestimate body fat in older adults who have lost muscle because its formula assumes a certain amount of muscle for each height. If you have lost muscle due to aging or lack of exercise, you will have more of your weight stored as fat. This means your BMI might indicate that you are in the normal range when in fact you have too much fat.

Given these flaws, in June 2023, the American Medical Association suggested that BMI, commonly used to categorize a person as underweight, normal weight, overweight, or obese based on weight and height does not help directly assess the effects of body fat mass on medical conditions such as hypertension and cardiovascular diseases for an individual. BMI does not take into account the impact of comorbidities, lifestyle issues, gender, ethnicity, familial conditions, and aging on one's health. Yet another reason that BMI is inaccurate is the influence of eating disorders on fat accumulation. These flaws suggest that there is a need to reevaluate the supposed link between obesity and insulin resistance that is often cited as the cause of Type 2 diabetes.

Are you ready to be honest about your weight?

To avoid Type 2 diabetes, your goal must be to take back control of your body and rediscover your authentic weight. You know when your weight is right for you because your brain knows when your fat cells are not full and your blood is not full of fatty acids and glucose. Obviously, you can also look in the mirror and see whether you are carrying layers of fat in your abdomen, hips, or buttocks. If so, you need to be honest with yourself and admit you would be healthier if you lost weight.

Regardless of where you land on a standard height/weight table or BMI chart, let your brain tell you the truth. Your health risks, particularly for diabetes, are related ultimately to how much of your weight is in your blood in the form of fat or glucose and how much of it is in your fat cells.

If you are unable to figure out what your authentic weight is, a good rule of thumb is that it is approximately the body weight you had when you were in your mid-20s, provided your blood sugar and triglyceride levels were within normal range at that time. That is the age at which you probably reached your full height, and your bones reached their maximum density. Any weight gain you experienced since that age will reflect the increase in pounds you have added over time due to storing fat and/or building muscle. (Note: for most people, as they age, weight gain is due to storing fat, not building muscle!)

Lose weight slowly

As you reconnect with your authentic weight, don't pressure yourself into believing you must lose extra pounds *quickly*, even if your blood sugar is high. If you think about it, you probably gained weight slowly over many years. There is no reason to think your body needs to lose it any faster than you gained it. Putting pressure on yourself to lose weight also tends to make you believe you should join a third-party weight loss program or go on a special diet. Neither of these is a worthwhile solution.

I suggest that setting a goal to lose just one pound per week is sufficient and appropriate. The value of losing weight slowly is that you can see what works best for you and is most successful at changing your eating habits, reducing side effects, and ensuring you can sustain your new weight for the longest period of time.

What counts most is seeing a downward trend in your weight week by week, month by month, until you arrive at your authentic weight. In addition, losing weight slowly gives your internal power-generating systems time to get used to the change in fuel usage (from burning fatty acids back to burning glucose), and it helps you maintain your skin elasticity without the danger of developing the sagging that occurs from rapid weight loss.

An effective way to lose weight after you binged and gained a pound or two

Are you going to an upcoming birthday celebration, wedding, or dinner party with friends, or a business meeting with lots of food and drink? If so, don't be surprised to see your weight go up by a few pounds or more after a celebration.

In fact, no matter how careful you are, it's likely you will experience weight gain on many occasions during the year, either from excess food intake or from energy-containing drinks. Therefore, it is imperative that you have a plan of action to deal with such occasions, preferably as soon as you notice how much exactly you have gained above your "authentic weight"—the weight your intuition tells you is right for your body.

Here is my recommendation. After any weight gain, for the next few days, your main meals should consist of salads made with a wide variety of vegetables. Start with a mix of greens of your choice, then add tomatoes, cucumbers, avocados, carrots, radishes, turnips, tender beetroots, bell peppers, both green and bulb onions, and other desirable items. Add small amounts of meat or cheese if desired. Change the combination from one meal to the next. Eat the salad without any dressing, the reason being so you can taste each nutrient without interference from any other flavor in the dressing. Using farm fresh, seasonal vegetables will give you the flavor as nature intended. I suggest that you avoid using items such as tomatoes that were selectively bred to increase sugar content.

Severely limit any grains or grain-flour products during these days because these are the main carriers of calories that add excess weight to your body if not burned immediately. Continue this pattern of eating until you have reduced your weight to the previous level.

A special note for women about losing weight

The worst way to lose weight is to focus on fixing your body image (an external motivation), rather than on getting in touch with your authentic weight (an internal motivation). This problem is especially true among women in our society. The desire for attention and acceptance by fellow humans, especially those who are considered "better" than you in appearance, is embedded in human nature. But in a society that uses the physical figure as the defining feature of female attractiveness, a media industry that promotes the feminine body appearance as the key to being appealing to others, and a weight loss industry constantly promoting "easily achievable" targets, too many women are fixated on body weight as the benchmark to feel happy and confident.

In my view, the bigger tragedy is that body appearance for women is fast becoming a multi-generational problem. A young girl growing up today in a household with a mother who herself has failed to maintain an authentic body weight may be lectured to about not gaining weight. The mother, unable to look at the reasons for her own failure, may be motivated by a desire to spare her daughter the frustration, humiliation, and feeling of helplessness that came with her own repeated attempts at weight maintenance. But that mother's nagging can have a psychological impact on her daughter.

The daughter, full of youthful energy and confidence, then tries to get support from her most trustworthy source, her peers, many of whom may be in the same situation. Collectively, they look for guidance from the most accessible source of information — the media, which perpetuates stereotypical female body images without any medical science or health reasons to support their claims. As these young girls grow to maturity, they tend to experience the same results as their mothers because they never learned anything meaningful about weight maintenance other than how they are supposed to look. The mothers never discuss with their daughters the more important topics related to health and weight for lifelong happiness rather than superficial perceptions of external beauty and appearance.

This cycle, as usual, continues as young girls become grown women and start their own families. Fearful of gaining weight and aware of the difficulty of maintaining authentic body weight based not only on their own experience but that of their mothers, these women tend to repeat the same pattern of focusing on external beauty with their own daughters.

This is a vicious multi-generational cycle that I believe requires attention and action by the medical community. We need more medical professionals to promote the body's natural regulatory mechanisms about food, teaching moms and daughters to recognize and respect when they are hungry and when they are satiated. Without such guidance, we will continue to have generations of mothers who teach their daughters what they should look like based on their own failed experiences and expectations of beauty. Girls, in turn, will continue to feel pressure to disconnect from their own natural control mechanisms of food intake in favor of media and stereotyped cultural images of beautiful women who are held out as models of appearance and lifestyle — while teaching them nothing about health and longevity.

How to return to your authentic weight

By far the best way to return to your authentic weight is to restrict your intake of certain food groups, particularly carbohydrates, added sugars, and salt.

Let me emphasize one point: it doesn't matter how fast you lose weight, as long as you do it in a way that helps you reduce your blood sugar. If you are genetically programmed to store a lot of fat in your body, it may be difficult for you to significantly reduce your body weight anyway. So for you, the only real choice is to adjust the quantity and type of foods you eat to lower blood sugar. This is enough to lose some weight and it is also the primary action you need to take to reverse your Type 2 diabetes.

Unfortunately, our personal habits and cultural environment both can have a powerful negative influence on the food quantities and choices we make in eating. We live in a culture where food is cheap and plentiful. We inhabit a body that is designed to store lots of fat. Capitalist food companies heavily promote cheap fast-food meals that look good and appeal to our taste. The medical community as a whole does not have consensus strong enough to undertake a national or global campaign to halt the pandemic of Type 2 diabetes.

In the end, it is up to you individually and your ability to respect your body, to seek to reconnect with your authentic weight, and to live a long, healthy life.

Will exercise help you lose weight?

Many people rely on exercise to lose weight. It is true that during exercise, muscles can absorb glucose without the presence of insulin and cause lowering of your blood sugar.

However, my position is that while exercise may help you lower your blood sugar, it often does not help most people to lose weight, simply because the amount of exercise you need to burn more calories than you consume in an average day is beyond possibility for most people.

I am not suggesting you do not exercise, as it serves an important role in conditioning your lungs, heart, and muscles. But reducing grains significantly and limiting your overall food consumption are steps which are far more beneficial if you are seriously interested in losing weight and reversing Type 2 diabetes. See Appendix 4 for more information about the real role of exercise in your health.

MAINTAIN YOUR AUTHENTIC WEIGHT: PAYING ATTENTION TO THE HUNGER SENSATION

IT CAN BE assumed with certainty that one cannot accumulate body fat while fasting. It can also be assumed that to keep on storing fat, one has to keep on eating energy-containing (high calorie) nutrients in excess of what the body can burn, no matter the nature of food consumed. Somewhere in between these two extremes is where your consumption of food should be. But how can you assess that?

The answer is: you must begin paying attention to and listening to your hunger signals. The desire to acquire nutrients — the hunger sensation — is present in all living things. How you respond to this natural signal will determine whether you are accumulating fat or not. Paying attention to your true hunger signals requires reconnecting with the vital messages that your brain gives you about hunger based on its ability to monitor your nutrient needs and to measure your nutrient intake.

Your brain has the same remarkable capability of monitoring your nutrient needs and taking inventory of your nutrient intake as it does of monitoring every element of your life. Just as your brain can evaluate your surroundings and warn you of danger, or listen closely to a symphony and pick out the piccolo part, or feel an itch in your lower back when you are giving a speech to an audience, it can detect the nutrient needs of every cell in your body and determine what foods you need to consume to provide those nutrients.

Distinguishing real hunger signals from other reasons you eat

What causes the brain to generate the hunger sensation? I have studied this topic for more than 25 years and suggest that there is a lot of misunderstanding about hunger. Here are some theories about why we feel hunger that I believe are incorrect:

1. The body is programmed to store a certain amount of fat that you can use for energy rather than by continuously eating. Since fat is created and taken apart on a continuous basis, could the total quantity of fat falling below a certain threshold level be responsible for the brain generating the sensation of hunger?

I don't think so, because if this were true, your sensation of hunger should stop once your fat stores are above a certain level and not resume until they fall below that threshold. That could take a long time, in which case humans would only eat every few days. For example, if you gained one pound of fat in the past week, one might think you wouldn't need to feel hunger until that that extra fat is used up. Conversely, if you lost several pounds of fat in a month, one might think you'd be eating continuously until that fat store is replenished to the threshold level. Both do not happen.

2. Might the sensation of hunger occur when the level of fat cir-
    culating in your body (in the bloodstream and fluids around
    cells) has gotten too low? This too is unlikely because the
    amount of circulating fat is small compared to the total fat in
    the body. Stored fat quickly converts to fatty acids that can be
    reconstituted by the liver into circulating fat. So there should
    be no need to eat simply to increase the amount of fat circulat-
    ing in the body.

3. A third theory for hunger is that when our storage of fat is low,
    it causes a messenger of some type to be released to notify the
    brain that we need more nutrition. It is true that fat cells actu-
    ally do secrete a small protein called *leptin* that has been iden-
    tified as a potential messenger candidate. However, nothing
    about leptin molecules in their amount, structure, or function
    has been linked to causing the hunger sensation to be gener-
    ated in most individuals.

4. A fourth possible cause of hunger relates to the glucose
    reserve in the body, which is limited to less than about 120
    grams of glycogen in the liver and about the same in mus-
    cles. These stores can be rapidly depleted during the period
    between meals. Therefore, might the hunger sensation be sig-
    naling the brain that we need to restore the glucose reserve
    in the body?

Again, this is unlikely. If low blood sugar is the cause of the hunger
sensation, then why do people with diabetes feel hunger even when
their blood sugar level is far higher than normal? One might argue
that diabetics have a lower level of glucose inside their cells or that
their sugar metabolism is defective, so they cannot be representative
of the general population. However, even people who do not have

diabetes feel the sensation of hunger when their blood sugar level is artificially kept high using a glucose drip into the vein.

5. Could the hunger sensation be generated by the arrival in the brain of a hormone released by the stomach or another part of the gastrointestinal tract? *Ghrelin,* a hormone released by cells in the stomach, can increase the intensity of hunger. But to date no one has identified a hormone that *initiates* the sensation of hunger or even a mechanism that activates the release of this hormone.

———

None of these explanations for hunger appear adequate or correct. I suggest that the answer relates to the fact that our brain acts as a "nutritional regulatory" system. The brain has an enormous capability of tracking the level of nutrients in our body, right down to the cellular level. The power of the brain to monitor and track your nutritional needs is no less extraordinary than the capacity of the brain to recall an incident that happened to you 30 or 40 years ago, to tell the muscles in your hand how to coordinate with your eye to play ping pong, or to recall the words and phonetics that allow you to speak one or more languages.

Given this, I contend that the hunger sensation is generated when the brain detects a critical depletion not just of glucose but also of many key nutrients essential for the normal functioning of the cells of your body. This is why even diabetics, who have high blood sugar, feel hunger. The brain, being the command center of our nutritional regulatory system, knows when many other key nutrients will soon be lacking (in addition to glucose).

Just as the brain detects an insufficiency of water in cells and bodily fluids and tells you that you are thirsty, it signals you to feel hunger when it detects that other needed nutrients are about to fall below optimum levels. This explains why you can feel the sensation of hunger at unpredictable intervals of time, even within a short time after eating, if not enough of some nutrient your body needed has been consumed.

The implications of listening to your brain's signals about hunger are important if you truly want to change your eating habits. Any time you are tempted to eat, first stop yourself and become aware and mindful of your hunger: is it real? Is your brain sending you signals that feel like you need nutrition? Or are you eating for other reasons — such as stress, habit, or peer pressure?

Listen closely and your brain also tells you what to eat

After getting a true hunger signal, how do we manage to get the nutrients that our brain has identified as lacking? Is it that we randomly choose what to eat based on what is in the pantry, what restaurants are nearby, or who we are with?

The answer is, your brain does attempt to guide you towards the right foods either through the unconscious decisions you make about what to eat — or via conscious cravings you have for specific foods. The brain has learned from your past eating habits and knows which foods will provide you with the missing nutrients. It has correlated the information stored in memory of foods you have already eaten and their nutrient components. These correlations began forming at the beginning of your life and continue to be made on an ongoing basis, building a database of nutrient-food correspondences that the brain uses to guide you.

In effect, the brain's regulatory system tracks your food and fluid intake during each meal and compares it, when possible, to the nutrients received from past experiences with the same foods. Your brain knows what nutritional value you get from a hamburger, a spaghetti dinner, a bowl of wonton soup, a burrito, chicken curry, or whatever foods are in your cultural background.

This capability of the brain is no different than how a toddler can listen to the same story or music over and over and the child's brain learns the words so that he or she can complete the story or song when listening to it later. In the same way, your brain becomes a databank of foods and their nutritional values — and pushes you to desire certain edibles when you need their nutrients.

Consider all those times when you find yourself asking, "What should I have for dinner tonight?" and an answer pops into your head without any trouble: "I need some meat," or "I feel like having some cheese tonight," or "Tonight's a good night for chicken and a salad." That is your brain telling you what nutrients it needs because it knows what nutrients those foods provide.

These messages are different for each person, of course, reflecting their past eating experiences, cultural background, and food preferences. The brain guides each of us first towards foods from which it knows it can obtain the necessary nutrients. For instance, onions, garlic, rice, and curry are meaningful sources of nutrients for some people and their brain will desire foods containing them. For others, these items will seem unpleasant to their brain, which prefers meat, salad, and potatoes because it knows their nutritional value.

Of course, this doesn't mean that people cannot enjoy new foods. That said, for most of history, humans have had very limited choices of food. In many ways, our modern world's access to so many foods offering an enormous variety of nutrients is an evolutionary leap. Each time we try a new food item or recipe, the brain updates its database, adding the new item and the nutrients it supplies to its inventory. This is why it's easy to enjoy new foods from other cultures yet begin craving them as much as foods you grew up with when you feel hungry.

The body needs many types of nutrients

The body needs many nutrients for normal functioning. Science has identified 118 nutrients that are used at some time for human health. No one knows with certainty how much of each of these the body needs or how we derive them from the foods we eat. That is why I always suggest eating a wide variety of foods to ensure you have the opportunity to ingest as many of these nutrients as possible. It is also why I do not believe in fixed diets or third-party programs that supply you with your meals.

Only your brain can tell you what you need to eat. Hunger is ultimately the only sensation the body can generate to make sure that you consume all needed nutrients. This also means, however, that the brain appears to have a natural inclination to acquire any nutrients the body needs, even if eating results in consuming other nutrients you do not immediately need.

My view is that the brain's signals to us about hunger and its attempt to steer us towards certain foods could be linked to the fact that the body needs to be able to utilize all available nutrients and this requires many agents around to absorb, transport, and break them down. In the end, the biology of digestion and nutrient absorption is far from being completely understood. It is likely that there are many interactions between nutrients that we are not yet aware of. I suggest that a lot of further study about nutrient interaction is needed.

Meanwhile, there is no denying that hunger enhances the intensity of your enjoyment. When you start your meal in a state of hunger, chances are your body needs multiple nutrients. Some may be needed only in minute quantities, while others require larger amounts.

When you are hungry, your brain creates a greater intensity of response to each bite of food, which you experience as enjoyment, based on the signals coming from your mouth, taste buds, and smell receptors. The amount of time your senses come into contact with nutrient molecules is much more important in experiencing enjoyment than the quantity passing through the mouth.

In summary, when you get hungry, to eat healthy, all you have to do is to become more aware of the intensity of your enjoyment, as your brain's pleasure sensation indicates the nutrients needed at that time.

MAINTAIN YOUR AUTHENTIC WEIGHT: LISTENING TO THE SIGNALS OF SATIATION

WE JUST EXPLORED the hunger sensation — what it is, why you become hungry and how your brain appears to guide you to select foods that have nutrients the body needs. Now you may wonder: Does the brain also tell you when to stop eating?

The answer is yes, there are also signals of satisfaction that are generated subconsciously and automatically. Like hunger signals, these "satiation" signals are highly dependent on your body's nutritional status — do you need more nutrients, or do you have enough after eating?

At some meals, you may need multiple nutrients and can eat a large quantity of food until your brain recognizes that you have consumed all the nutrients necessary. At other meals, you will be quickly satiated after you have eaten only a small amount, either because you needed only a small number of nutrients, or the food you consumed was very rich in the needed nutrients — or even in some cases, the food you consumed did not have any of the needed nutrients.

Information regarding the nature and concentration of nutrients is generated from the moment food enters the mouth till waste products exit the body. How this information is collected, relayed to the brain's control center, and acted upon will determine the quantity of food you would ideally consume during each meal. The most significant signals telling you to stop eating are those generated when food encounters sensors located at the point of entry into the body — your mouth.

Signals from the mouth

Your mouth plays a significant role not only in the enjoyment of eating, but also in giving you cues to stop eating. You may not realize that these two roles that your mouth plays are actually closely associated. The enjoyment of eating starts with the feel of a bite of food you just took. The tactile experience of eating comes from the texture of the food in the mouth, not from the feeling of fullness in the mouth from a single large bite of food. Textures of foods differ, so the more you chew each bite multiple times, the more it adds to the tactile experience and pleasure of eating.

With this in mind, I suggest that chewing is an integral part in the acquisition of needed nutrients, and it relieves the hunger sensation. Most importantly though, it also prevents you from overeating if you pay attention. The act of chewing breaks food into smaller particles, releasing nutrients in your mouth. The movement of your lower teeth by the jaw muscles also registers inside your brain and adds to the tactile experience of eating. When you pay attention to your food during a meal, and chew slowly, it gives your brain the time to recognize the nutrients in the food by the signals generated by your taste and smell sensors. These sensors are ideally located to assist your brain in accomplishing the tasks of monitoring incoming nutrients in your food.

The key principle here is to heighten your awareness of both the sensory experience (the smells and tastes of the food) and the mechanical action of chewing. Both are critical to knowing when to stop eating. By paying attention to the sensations created in the mouth during the act of chewing, the brain has an open channel of communication to inform you what to do next: continue eating or stop. As you eat and start to fill yourself, the combinations of signals from your taste and smell sensors cause your brain to respond by creating a drop in the intensity of flavor of the food. This deliberate act by the brain helps regulate your food intake. When your intensity of enjoying what you eat drops, you need to put down your fork. That is the signal from your brain to stop eating.

How much food do you really need?

Rather than paying attention to the process of eating (tasting and chewing), most people eat automatically according to the culture they grew up in. In many societies, the typical pattern of eating includes three meals per day of varying sizes, plus morning and afternoon snacks, and perhaps an added dessert. If you were not reading this book, you might continue eating this exact way for the rest of your life, following the same routines you learned in childhood, which are reinforced by our highly scheduled culture, organized around work hours and school for kids and adopted by millions of families throughout the world.

But think about it:

- Do you need all this nutrition?
- Are you listening to your brain's hunger signals?
- Do you know what your hunger signals are and how to respond to them properly so you do not over-consume energy nutrients (calories) your body does not need?

Paying attention to your enjoyment of eating

My explanation of our regulatory mechanism of nutrient intake — based on our sensory experiences of taste, smell, and chewing — is applicable to humans of all ages — infants, toddlers, children, and adults. Our nutritional regulatory system is no different than how our other senses prompt our brain to react to stimuli.

For example, while looking at a painting, your brain understands colors of varying intensity and the lines of demarcation between them. When listening to music, your brain can differentiate the rhythm, loudness, and tempo of notes from different sources of instruments. This in-the-moment enjoyment of the painting and music is possible because signals travel to and between neurons in the brain at speeds faster than 250 mph (which is a very fast speed considering the small space inside our heads).

In the very same way, our brain acts as a regulatory system that uses the senses to determine the nutritional value of what we eat. As toddlers, we would not be able to develop an appetite for foods without having a natural mechanism to monitor the nutrient needs in the body. Toddlers would also be unable to consume adequate amounts of food for normal growth and development without a natural mechanism to measure incoming nutrients and assess how much is needed and what is missing. In other words, the hunger mechanism is built into the human brain.

Evidence for the presence of an innate mechanism in infants and children for regulating food intake was actually established decades ago. Effectively, the human species would not exist if the brain were not helping us determine what and how much to eat.

Being able to enjoy your food requires that you keep your taste and smell receptors healthy. Nature does its part by replacing taste cells every few days. Nerve cells that detect smell sensation are replaced at the rate of one percent each day. It is your duty to keep these sensors in proper working order through oral hygiene, including brushing your teeth. It is important to stay hydrated as well to ensure you have a good salivary flow.

OVERCOME YOUR TENDENCIES TO OVEREAT

YOU PROBABLY love food. It's hard to resist a good meal. But until you began reading this book, you might not have thought much about food as a collection of molecules containing the nutrients your cells need to function. You know, of course, that food provides your body with energy and vitamins and minerals, but what has been missing in your understanding is the impact of what you eat at the micro-level, where food breaks down into single molecules of energy nutrients and essential nutrients. You probably also never thought about your brain as a regulatory system that monitors and tracks your nutrient intake — using your taste sensors, smell receptors, the sensations in your mouth, the hormones in your stomach and intestines, and the levels of glucose and nutrients in your blood as it flows through the brain.

So if these sophisticated mechanisms have developed in humans, why do so many people overeat? Why doesn't the brain help us completely regulate our sensations of hunger and satisfaction such that we never gain weight, never consume too much food that floods our bloodstream with glucose, and never develop high blood sugar and diabetes? I suggest two potential reasons for you to consider.

Eating when there is no real hunger signal

We have discussed the role of hunger sensation in selecting food items containing nutrients needed in the body at the time of each meal. However, what happens if you are eating not in response to a true hunger signal? The brain, not expecting information on incoming nutrients, will not be able to help you regulate the quantity consumed at that time. How many times have you consumed food as part of a celebration, even when not hungry? How often do you nibble something because you are bored and have nothing to do? Do you use eating to relieve stress and anxiety? Do you go get some food to avoid work? Do you stop for a snack so as not to go home for some reason?

The factors that fuel our desire to eat even when we are not hungry are likely quite complex and intermixed with many elements of our psychological makeup, cultural background, and family dynamics. But these are all factors that you must gain control of if you find yourself eating when not hungry, gaining weight, or if your doctor reports that you have high blood sugar.

Think about this. As an infant, toddler, and very young child, you probably did not eat when you were not hungry. Most very young children are completely in touch with their hunger and satisfaction signals. They only eat when hunger drives them to do so, and then only as much as they can handle.

I suggest that non-hunger eating begins as a temporary and occasional accident, done without recognizing its long-range significance. It then repeats a few times until it becomes a habit.

In most people, it first occurs as incidental to other events or situations, such as a family picnic or holiday dinner, a chance meeting with a friend, or an unplanned spur-of-the-moment meal with someone. It is not a deliberate act of overeating, but a random occurrence.

However, the more these "extra" eating events occur in one's early life, the more repetition reinforces the brain to make connections between eating and enjoyment. Whether you are hungry or not, if food is available and appealing, you learn to feel it is okay to eat it. You may sense that it's not appropriate to be eating when you are not hungry, and even those who cared for you during your childhood might have told you not to do it. But little by little, you begin to rationalize that since food serves a good purpose, eating just a little bit without being hungry can't be that bad. And when you are young, your high level of activity may prevent you from gaining much weight. The enjoyment of discovering new foods and the pleasure of eating them eventually overcomes your natural inclination to wait for the sensation of hunger.

In this way, you begin to establish a behavior of eating when simply stimulated by the sight, smell, or even just the thought of food rather than by your body's hunger signals, just because you like the feeling of enjoyment. The connection between food and enjoyment is stored in your memory and expresses itself without any conscious or deliberate effort. Smelling food cooking, walking into a colorful supermarket, passing by a restaurant — all these trigger in you a pleasurable feeling caused by the release of *dopamine*, a neuro-hormone that prompts you to want food. You look forward to enjoying a variety of good quality, tasty foods.

Once this rationale is established, even your growing awareness of potential adverse long-term consequences such as weight gain, high blood sugar, high blood cholesterol, or high blood pressure may not be sufficient deterrents to modify your response to food. This is because the brain has difficulty connecting immediate behavior with long-term consequences. If the ill effects do not immediately follow the causal action, it is easy to rationalize a behavior. Your subconscious mind cannot make value judgments, deciding whether what you're doing is good or bad. It simply remembers and accepts what you have been doing and facilitates the execution of the established behavior. The behavior continues, even when the consequences are damaging.

This pattern of behavior is not unlike other unhealthy behaviors you might have cultivated in your life for pleasure, such as gambling, overworking, sex, or even accumulating wealth. Once you accept the activity as normal, it becomes difficult to stop repeating it over and over.

Eating too much based on factors other than satiation

In addition to eating when not hungry, you might overeat because you remain unaware of the signals to stop eating that your mouth or brain generate, or because of other factors. Here are several common causes of overeating.

The first is that you may overeat in the sense of consuming too much of the wrong food. This type of overeating can also begin unconsciously. While hunger triggers the conscious decision to initiate eating, your subconscious mind is not controlled by rational thought and is easily swayed to follow eating patterns you established long ago. For example, if as a child or teen, you repeatedly consumed fruit juice or soda in response to thirst, the subconscious mind can interpret the thirst sensation as a need for soda and not water. If you routinely had eggs, bacon, and biscuits, or a bowl full of cereal for breakfast when you grew up, the brain could create a craving for these in the morning even though the body does not need nutrients from these items. In effect, you may be hungry when you eat, but you consume too much of the wrong nutrients out of habit. This type of overnutrition can lead to weight gain and high blood sugar.

A second reason you may overeat could be that you rely too much on the sensation you receive from the stomach to tell you to stop eating. The problem with this is, the stomach normally has relatively little tone in its muscular wall, allowing it to expand and bulge progressively outward. Relying on the feeling of fullness to stop eating is like relying on the feeling of the fullness of a water balloon to determine when to stop putting in water. Because the balloon can stretch, you can put a lot of water in it before it gets full — a point that is almost impossible to know beforehand. In the same way, your stomach muscle can keep stretching to accommodate a large quantity of food — up to more than one liter in volume — before you feel full. Recall how you can feel completely stuffed at the end of a sumptuous meal, but if dessert you enjoy is available, you will still eat it.

You're able to do this because your stomach expands, and only when it reaches a certain stage of expansion do you finally stop eating. Rather than paying attention to the feeling of satisfaction during a meal, you become accustomed to waiting until you sense your stomach stretching almost to the point of discomfort before you decide to stop eating.

A third reason why you may overeat is that you are preoccupied and do not appreciate the sense of satisfaction generated by the control centers in your brain. It's natural to enjoy eating, but the key to regulating your food intake is to completely enjoy what you eat by focusing on the sensations you experience when you taste the food.

I am encouraging you to let your brain do its natural work of matching the intake of nutrients that pass through your mouth to the deficit of nutrients in your cells that the brain has already identified. If you are preoccupied with some other thought or action, your brain may not be focusing on recognizing the nutrients being consumed. This is because the conscious part of your brain can concentrate only on one activity at a time.

When you eat with focus, your conscious mind sees some uneaten food on your plate, which the subconscious mind has already determined has nutritional value. However, the conscious mind will try to listen to the signals coming from the brain indicating the degree of enjoyment and decide whether you are still in need of nutrients from that food. In this way, your conscious mind can control how much you eat.

However, if you are reading, watching TV, or performing an action while eating, your subconscious mind takes over and will encourage eating because it knows the food has nutritional value or is simply following past eating behaviors already programmed in your brain. Your subconscious mind cannot pay attention to the signals from your mouth indicating a decreasing enjoyment of the food. If the subconscious mind is programmed to stop eating only when the plate is empty or your stomach has expanded to a discomfort level, the result is likely to be excess consumption relative to your actual nutritional needs. In short, if you want to be confident in your ability to disregard food on your plate no matter how pleasing it looks or good it smells, you must engage your conscious mind during the meal you're eating. I call this "mindful eating."

A fourth reason for overeating is that your taste and smell receptors are unable to record the amount of nutrients passing through the mouth. For example, when you eat food that is soft and requires hardly any chewing, such as rice or mashed potatoes, you are likely to swallow it immediately. When you drink blended or pureed foods, you also would have trouble deciding how much to take in to feel satisfied, because you are forced to swallow the liquid before your brain can ascertain the nutrient content of each mouthful. On the other hand, when you slowly and deliberately chew your food, you not only enjoy what you are consuming, but you will also feel satisfied with less food compared to the amount swallowed without your chewing it.

Finally, a fifth reason for overeating without paying attention to your satiation signals is that we now have an increasing availability of food items produced with ingredients in concentrations higher than that found in natural foods. The brain's control mechanisms, designed to regulate our intake of nutrients, are based on the concentrations of nutrients found in nature. When you eat processed foods full of starches, fat, salt, sugars, artificial flavorings, and chemical ingredients, your brain cannot assess when you should stop eating. You effectively become addicted to the taste, smells, and textures of those foods to the point of preferring them to natural foods.

Humans were not designed to overeat

From a biological standpoint, the human body was not constructed to overeat on a consistent basis and gain excess weight to the point of causing high blood sugar and diabetes. The body doesn't need to store more than a small amount of fat. The purpose of our digestive system and fat cells is to capture nutrients we might need on an immediate "just-in-time" basis. Similarly, the brain's regulatory system was designed to produce feelings of satisfaction and pleasure when we consume food that supplies our body with the nutrients it needs for our daily activities.

What is happening to humans in much of the world today is an exposure to an endless quantity and variety of foods that activate our excitement and pleasure. It is biologically natural to feel a desire to eat these foods. But as we begin eating too much of those foods, as well as too much of the wrong foods that are mass produced in our industrial food complex — e.g., grain-based carbohydrates with added sugars, fats, and salt — we reinforce behaviors that repeatedly trigger the pleasure response system of the brain. We thus begin overeating regularly because it induces these familiar pleasurable feelings. We are then no longer content to feel the enjoyment that comes with eating just enough to feel satisfied relative to our true hunger.

Evidence of this "food bonanza" phenomenon abounds in societies where high blood sugar and diabetes are rapidly increasing. In these cultures, restaurants often serve extremely large portions of carbohydrate-based foods compared to the amount a normal human needs for nutrition in a single meal. Some restaurants even make an entire business out of offering people expansive "all you can eat" specials, as if to challenge them to overeat until they are bloated and sick.

Sugared drinks and food products packed with carbohydrates and salt are packaged and marketed in ways to make us associate them with happiness, sexuality, success, and good times. Even when people cook at home, they have trained themselves through habit to serve large portions and eat everything on their plate regardless of the satiation signals they may receive from their brain. In addition, they take pride in showing who can provide the most variety of foods to entertain family and friends.

People in many societies, not just the US, are losing control of the natural human mechanisms to eat healthy and enjoy their food. We are succumbing to powerful external forces that are motivated by profit — the food industry and advertisers and marketers of food products. Diabetes existed only as a rare human condition for thousands of years, a biological phenomenon based on bodily chemistry. However, with weight gain and obesity now affecting an estimated one-third of the entire global population, it is clear that factors outside of normal human biological phenomena are driving epidemic levels of Type 2 diabetes. Nothing short of a revolutionary approach can reverse this epidemic.

TAKE CONTROL OF YOUR EATING HABITS

I S IT POSSIBLE to regain control of your eating habits? Fortunately, the answer is yes. It is obvious that if you have been diagnosed as diabetic, you have not yet understood on a deep level how to control your eating behaviors. This step will teach you how to achieve this control.

Many of you may feel skeptical about trying yet another approach if you have experienced failures with other "lifestyle changing" attempts. But I invite you to allow this book to be your inspiration to finally take your life back.

Whatever your reaction, I want to help you feel confident that you can regain control of your eating habits. Think about this: how can anyone else tell you what to eat on a daily basis if you yourself can't know which nutrients or how much of each your body needs when you start eating? In other words, *your own brain is the only location with the precise information of your body's needs.*

If you begin to reflect on what you have learned so far in this book — the real cause of diabetes, the serious impact that eating a high grain-based diet has, and how your brain's nutritional regulatory system can help you listen closely to its signals of hunger and satisfaction — you can make meaningful changes in how you eat to reverse your diabetes.

Keep in mind that even though high blood sugar can be reversed in just 8 weeks, making and sustaining long-term changes in your eating behaviors may take months of practice and you will need to keep at it, even if your blood sugar level has been normalized.

Recognize that changing lifelong eating habits is possible

Evolution did not create humans who require three meals a day plus a few snacks and desserts. Most of us are conditioned to eat and enjoy food from the day we are born. Our eating habits are developed when we are children and reinforced as we age, so changing them as adults becomes a mental struggle against decades of ingrained behavior around food. Our eating patterns and habits become so natural, so automatic, and so unchangeable that we do not even recognize them as being culturally determined or under our complete control.

Recognize that your eating habits began in your childhood. During the first year of life, you tripled your body weight. Your parents, grandparents, uncles, aunts, and other relatives and family friends encouraged your efforts at eating, marveled at your achievements, and adored your bodily appearance. This began your love affair with food — and with good reason, as you wouldn't have survived infancy without that nourishment.

After the first year of life, you stopped gaining weight at the same rate as you did in your first year, because nature has built-in control mechanisms to match your food intake more closely to the growing needs of your body. This was the period when your cells needed nutrients to build your organs and expand your brain cells, and your eating habits were dictated by your body, not by the conditioned behaviors of the adults around you.

Even by five years of age, most children still do not eat according to family habits or culturally determined behaviors. If you have ever watched a young child eat, you know that they eat only what they want and when they want. They will stubbornly resist parents pushing them to eat at prescribed times or to eat what's on the dish. And if they eat excess food during one meal, they compensate for it with reduced intake during subsequent meals because their brain knows how much nourishment they need.

In effect, young children literally learn to listen closely to the signals (or intuitions) from the brain telling them when they are hungry and when they are satisfied. They intuitively eat to stay at their authentic weight.

As they grow up, however, most children eventually begin falling into patterns highly influenced by their family's eating behaviors, their taste preferences, and their culture. Recall your own experience. It is likely that you began having meals at the same time your parents did. You ate the food choices for your meals that were given to you — whether it was meat and potatoes in some families, Chinese food in others, or vegetarian in still others.

But the teen years were also the age that, like your peers, you may have started to expand your tastes as you experimented with foods you saw on TV, in advertisements, at friend's homes, and in the movies — cereals, fancy cupcakes, chocolate-covered anything, and perhaps even novel items for the very brave — sushi, Vietnamese *Pho,* fancy Italian pastas, Moroccan couscous, and many other ethnic specialties full of rice, wheat, and other grains.

This expanded diet doesn't usually impact teens though. Active teenagers can usually eat to their heart's content — even if it is full of carbs, sugar, and fat — and still maintain their weight within a range of a pound or two. Most teens do not become prediabetic, because their metabolism utilizes all the food they eat. Their bodies are lengthening bones and building muscle mass. Even if they keep some fat in storage, it is quickly used to produce energy when they need it between meals.

The problem for most teens today, however, is that their eating habits are being increasingly assaulted by the modern world and the foods being manufactured and advertised. We see millions of young people falling prey to unhealthy snack foods and meal choices that are aggressively marketed to them on TV and online. Lured by these products, children are losing their body's natural ability to remain at their authentic weight at increasingly early ages. Millions more children around the world will grow into adults with eating habits that push them into diabetes.

Your eating habits pursue you into adulthood

If you are an adult with elevated blood sugar reading this book, whatever poor eating habits you developed during your childhood and teen years have likely persisted into adulthood. You probably continue to enjoy eating foods that remind you of pleasurable experiences and memories of good times from your past. It is also likely that you adopted several unhealthy eating habits as you aged, based on other factors, such as the following:

- You may have developed a taste for eating a lot of certain types of ethnic foods whose flavors and spices are different from what you grew up with.
- You may eat between meals because you are stressed out.
- You may eat too much at dinnertime because you skipped lunch during your busy workday and now enjoy sitting around the table talking to your family or guests while constantly eating.
- You may have added alcohol into your mealtimes or between them without considering the extra calories that alcoholic beverages add to your daily intake.

- And as you got older, you may have simply become conditioned to eat at certain times of the day, whether you are hungry or not.
- Yet another behavior you may have acquired is chewing too fast. This limits the duration of time available for your taste and smell sensors to detect incoming nutrients and inform your brain's control centers to determine when to send the satiation signal.

When all these factors are combined, it is easy to see how you can lose touch with your authentic body weight and fail to listen to your brain's messages about hunger and satisfaction. Instead of paying attention to the signs that you are truly hungry, your other habits and behaviors take over.

Paradoxically, I am convinced that most people are completely aware when they are eating unhealthy foods and overeating. They hear that little voice in their brain telling them to stop eating so much, or to eat something healthier, because the brain has been monitoring their nutritional needs. But they ignore that voice because other voices in the brain assure them that they will derive pleasure from other foods or from continuing to eat.

I have news for you. *You will not reverse Type 2 diabetes unless you begin to listen to the voice in your head about how much you should truly eat.* You must alter your dietary habits and return to your authentic weight. For many of you, this means emptying your fat cells as much as possible, as well as taking back control of your food intake.

How to break old patterns to change your eating behavior

Throughout your life, each time you have eaten something, your brain has received millions of signals from your taste and smell receptors.

Each experience has produced specific connections between nerve cells in your brain to form pathways about eating, which have been strengthened through repeated use. The way you have been eating has effectively been "hardwired" and solidified as a neural network in your brain. It has become self-sustaining and, more importantly, hard to change because it's not stored as a file that can easily be deleted.

It used to be thought that once the brain had established most of its connections during childhood, it would only change in response to aging. However, it has come to light that the brain has the ability to rewire itself to form new connections and learn different solutions to obtain a different result. This resourcefulness of the brain can be used to overcome an established behavior and accomplish a positive outcome.

Whenever you learn something, new nerve connections are established and consolidated. Unlearning something (such as an old habit) therefore requires weakening of the established connections between neurons. Because this work has to be done piecemeal, it takes time.

Luckily, the adult brain is reasonably accustomed to unlearning. If you ever moved homes or changed cities to study or work in a new city, you probably had to change your routines and habits. If you started living with someone, you had to rearrange millions of brain pathways to accommodate that person. Such unlearning requires "disconnecting" established neural paths and making new ones — one pathway after another and one network of neurons after another.

The point is, somewhere in your past, you have unlearned some things and learned new ones. You can do it again. The same unlearning and new learning can occur to retrain yourself about how and what you eat. To establish a new behavior pattern that promotes healthy eating, begin by finding ways to prevent activating the established pathways that promote unhealthy eating.

Here are some recommendations to begin unlearning your old habits by unravelling established pathways you have about food:

- Walk around your home and identify the areas and sights that test and break your control over food — and eliminate or modify them. For example, put all food in cabinets where it can't be seen.
- Buy food only using a prepared shopping list so you are not tempted to buy extra items on impulse.
- Pre-plan your meals and cook up and serve smaller portion sizes.
- Avoid locations that you associate with eating, such as food aisles in convenience stores, fast-food restaurants, stores serving free food samples, and vending machines that prompt you to buy food on impulse.
- Work on creating an environment that is not focused around food in your home. If pleasing sensations that are commonly paired with eating surround you, it's hard to deny the impulse to indulge. The sight and smell of sweets like ice cream, cookies, and cakes can stimulate the urge to eat, so don't bake desserts and don't stock ice cream in your freezer. The goal is to decrease temptation by reducing the sights, sounds, and smells of pleasing impulses.

Eating during celebrations, due to boredom and from stress

If you know or recognize that you sometimes eat not because of true hunger, but to take part in celebrations, due to boredom, or to cope with stress, it helps to have a detailed plan for dealing with those situations.

First, you may need to adjust your response to these events in general before you can change your pattern of eating. This is because your eating response is interconnected with your reactions to these situations in general, and thus runs through the many well-established and highly linked pathways in your brain. For example, de-emphasize the food so you can concentrate on the people and the occasion during celebrations. Find activities such as reading, learning a new skill, listening to music, talking to someone, meditating, taking a walk, gardening, etc., as substitutes for eating to deal with boredom and stress. You may need professional help to create new ways to deal with stress-related events.

Similarly, make sure that you end your meals based on satisfaction rather than on the sensation of fullness in the stomach or emptiness of the plate. Concentrate on enjoying what you eat. The best way to accomplish this is explained below.

Rediscover the eating behavior of your childhood

I wrote earlier that, for most people, their childhood eating habits were based on true hunger and satisfaction. You ate enough to grow and function but you did not overeat. Over time, however, your parents, the other people in your life, the environment in which you lived, the choices presented to you and your life experiences have all contributed to modifying your childhood eating behavior patterns.

Your mission to rediscover and maintain your authentic weight may get a psychological boost if you think of your journey as reestablishing the eating behavior of your childhood so that it matches your body's need for nutrients. This image can help you internalize the feeling that if your need for nutrients is not real, you should not be eating. If the need is minimal, ask yourself if you can wait until your brain evaluates the need relative to nutrients in storage and then generates the sensation of hunger.

I realize this is very difficult to do. In the modern world, advertising directly and indirectly involving food often creates the urge to eat. Your brain, instead of responding to nutrient needs, is tempted many times per hour to imagine the pleasure of eating.

Every day, you must make decisions about what to eat. When you eat out or eat at somebody's house, you have less choice about what to eat because you're eating off a menu or what the host has cooked. You must be alert when you decide to eat, choose the food you want to eat, and be aware during your meal to enjoy what you eat.

Just as a story is presented using groupings of different words, a behavior is formed by a series of nerve connections. To change the story line, you need to dismantle multiple parts, if not the whole, of the original word groupings and form different ones. Similarly, to change your behavior, you will have to destroy many established nerve connections and form new ones.

Be patient. This change will take time because of the strength of your brain's existing networks makes it easy to reactivate old connections and fall back into your former patterns. How much importance you give to the new way of eating will determine how effective you are at rewiring your brain. You must not only learn to do things that work but avoid falling back into previous behavior patterns that promote excess consumption.

Once you begin making a few major changes to modify the neural networks in your brain and delete old connections, you will be able to establish new pathways for a different behavior around eating within several weeks.

Making the behavior permanent may require months of practice. Repetition not only strengthens the connections between certain populations of neurons, but also makes it easier to activate them. If you reach a plateau in your progress, it's often a sign that the brain needs time to consolidate the changes already made before further ones can be accommodated.

Establishing a behavior pattern conducive to maintaining your authentic weight requires commitment and determination, but once the pattern is firmly established it becomes relatively easy to follow. By repeating your new behavior day after day, changes in your brain connections will become more refined and the new behavior more automatic.

A good snack to stave off hunger

There are times when you find it hard to stick to your commitment. For example, at the end of a long day at work, it is possible your neurons may be depleted of the neurochemicals needed to generate a disciplined behavior.

If that is the case, you could decide to postpone taking complete control and settle for a temporary state by eating a little bit of food even without the hunger sensation being triggered. I recommend that you keep a stash of nuts for these occasions. Fat-containing foods such as nuts speed the release of intestinal hormones faster than carbohydrate-based foods, so your hunger abates more quickly. If you are hungry for a snack, it is better to eat nuts rather than carbs such as chips.

Tapping into your willpower

You need to create a different way to initiate and complete food intake to begin forming new patterns about your eating behavior. Each action you perform in your life, including thinking about eating, requires the participation of thousands of nerve cells in the brain. When you start any action, those cells are already set to interpret signals in the way they have been programmed to do in your past. Changing your eating behavior, such as why you eat, what you eat, and more importantly how you eat, requires reprogramming nerve cells involved in the act.

In other words, you must relearn the meaning of eating. You may not have much control over the occurrence of sight, sound, smell, and random thought-related cues that trigger your desire to eat, especially in places beyond your own environment. But you can moderate the effect of these cues by changing the processing that happens in your brain after these sensory impulses are received. For this, your brain has to decide consciously to override your old, conditioned response. You must be able to tell yourself that the smell or sight of food does not mean you must eat it.

We commonly call the ability to resist something "willpower." You need willpower to resist eating when you're not hungry and only eat when you are. To generate willpower, you need to practice control over your impulse to eat. It is easier if you are already behaving in a disciplined way in other fields in your life.

Most everyone has willpower in something in their life they can tap into. If you get to your job every morning on time, you likely have willpower that you can apply to your eating behavior. If you clean your house every Saturday without fail, you have willpower. If you take a shower every day, you have willpower.

Your thoughts are the manifestation of your will. Thoughts can be the results of your will to act, or they can direct the will to form. It requires effort and training to keep your focus on beneficial thoughts. The good news is that an established thought process regarding eating can be modified based on reasoning driven by two important motivations.

The first is this. If you train yourself to eat better, you can avoid a lifetime of medications to lower sugar and fat levels, unwanted side effects of the medications, and the unavoidable suffering from the complications of diabetes. The second is the realization that you will feel and look better, become more active, and enjoy life far more by maintaining your authentic weight. Be aware that if your mind is preoccupied with thoughts of other pressing matters or inert with no sense of purpose, you may not feel the urgency to exercise your willpower.

What to do when you are dining out

Dining out at restaurants is challenging when you are trying to change your eating habits, especially cutting carbohydrates. If you go to a restaurant that puts a basket of bread on the table before you even order, remind yourself of your commitment to limit eating grains. Avoid going to restaurants that specialize in cuisines that encourage you to eat a lot of grain-flour foods such as sandwiches, pasta, pizza, and desserts. If you have some favorite restaurants that fit in this category, order items that contain the least amount of carbohydrates. Don't think that whole wheat or multigrain bread or pasta is better for you; it's still grain that produces voluminous amount of glucose that your body will need to store, and if your fat cells are still full, this will cause your muscle cells to continue the fatty acid burn switch.

Similarly, if you are invited to a friend's home and presented with a dish high in grain-based foods, show appreciation to the host and chef by eating some of the dish but not a large helping. Remember that you do not need to equate your gratitude with how much food you consume. This can be difficult in some cultures where hosts not only feel insulted if guests do not eat everything on their plate, but also encourage them to eat more than one serving.

Whether dining out with other people or at someone's home, here's one strategy that you might try, not only to help yourself but also to educate the people you love around you. Explain to your friends and family that you are seeking to change your eating habits based on what you learned in this book about the nutrients our bodies need, the linkage between grains and high blood sugar, and the growing risks of diabetes affecting people in all walks of life. Perhaps your family and friends will feel motivated to change their eating patterns with you.

Spread the word about the pandemic of diabetes and its consequences. In fact, if you participate in helping to build a natural movement to halt the pandemic of diabetes develops and the majority of people in the world begin altering their eating behavior, it will be an antidote to the powerful food industry that keeps on producing unhealthy foods and to the restaurants that serve large portions of carbohydrates and salty foods.

Prescribed diets and packaged foods

If you agree that the sensation of hunger represents the need to replenish nutrients your body's cells need, you can also understand the fact that you yourself have no idea of what specific nutrients the body is lacking at that time. This means no one else has a clue either. When you give the responsibility of determining what you eat and how much you eat to someone else, someone who has no intimate knowledge of your bodily needs, you lose the opportunity to retrain your brain. This is why nearly all third-party dieting and weight loss programs fail in the long run.

The same is true if you are tempted to use prepackaged diet foods or to follow instructions from one of the corporate weight loss management programs to help you accomplish your weight loss goals. If you rely on outside instructions and prepackaged foods, you may not be able to form new neural pathways that create new eating behaviors using real food. The moment you stop following the prescribed diet or using prepackaged foods and go back to eating on your own, you will likely revert to most of your old eating patterns — not chewing your food, not tasting the nutrients, not eating slowly and letting the signals from your mouth and nose reach the brain and notice the moment of satisfaction. This is why nearly all people who try a third-party weight loss program regain any weight they lost once they exit the program.

I hope this step has shown you that changing your eating behavior must involve consciously trying to alter the neural pathways in your brain. You need to establish and reinforce new connections in the brain that support the elements of conscious eating — chewing slowly, tasting your food, paying attention to the signals from your mouth, and so on. The best way to achieve and maintain your authentic weight and cut out excess food consumption is to learn this new eating behavior to replace your old one.

My recommendation is that you take responsibility for changing your own eating behavior. It is far better to prepare and eat your own food, so you can learn to eat right no matter what you consume. As I mentioned, I have published a cookbook, *The Diabetes-Free Cookbook and Exercise Guide*, to help people learn to prepare breakfasts, lunches, dinners, and snacks using healthy ingredients that are largely grain-free.

Developing the skills and ability to control your own eating can be done more easily by letting your internal regulatory system be in charge rather than some external system of food management or supplements. Doing it this way builds up your confidence in your ability to make your own food selections based on enjoyment. Your conscious mind can learn to concentrate on enjoying every morsel of food that you consume to meet the objective of adjusting the meal size. Your mealtime is your own to enjoy. Do not allow anyone to take that away from you.

UNDERSTAND THE FOODS YOU EAT

THE HUMAN BODY needs the same types of nutrients regardless of the environment it lives in. Humans have survived and still survive in cold weather climates, warm weather areas, jungles, prairies, islands, mountains, in houses floating on water, and inside houses made of ice or from rocks. In other words, all the nutrients the human body needs can be obtained from foods available in each of these locations, although packaged in different forms of carbohydrate, protein, fat, minerals, vitamins, and other yet unknown nutrients. The result is that all life forms, plants, animals, humans, etc., depend on foods available locally and seasonally, thanks to biodiversity and sunlight. Understanding how we depend on nature to acquire the nutrients we need in a timely fashion can help you select and consume various types of food.

The role of carbohydrates in human nutrition

Humans need some carbohydrates for functioning. Our cells use glucose, a carbohydrate, as their primary fuel. Dissolved glucose is always present in the blood and in the fluid around cells. The normal blood glucose concentration in a person who has not eaten a meal within the past three to four hours is 90 mg/dl. In a normal person, about an hour after a meal containing a large amount of carbohydrates — such as bread, pasta, rice, potatoes, or corn — the blood glucose level will seldom rise above 140 mg/dl because most of the glucose enters the cells of the body where it is used for energy. Glucose also remains in the fluid around cells, usually in the range of 75 to 95 mg/dl, though it can fluctuate in the short term between 20 and 1500 mg/dl without any harmful consequences. If the blood glucose level falls below one-half of normal, people usually experience a loss of mental functions — confusion, forgetfulness, and lack of analytic capabilities.

Carbohydrates in the form of *fructose* (fruit sugar) and *galactose* (milk sugars) are also necessary to perform specialized functions in cell membranes. For example, these sugars combine with protein or fat molecules that dangle outside cell walls and repel charged particles because of their negative charge. These combined structures attach themselves to carbohydrates protruding from other cells to maintain the cohesion of cells within an organ. These combined structures also act as receptors for binding hormones in cells and participate in our immune defense mechanisms by attacking bacteria in the blood, saliva, and tears.

The identification of your blood type as A, B, AB, or O is based on the presence of these structures on the red cell membrane. In addition, a special carbohydrate molecule is used in the construction of genes that reside inside the control center of each cell (the nucleus), and a variation of that molecule is used to manufacture the messenger that carries instructions from genes to workers in the cell.

But as I have pointed out, humans do not need so much glucose. We can derive our cellular fuel from fatty acids, produced from the fats we consume as well as from triglycerides that the liver produces from excess glucose produced in digestion. In climates that do not allow people to grow grains or have easy access to vegetables, the liver can produce glucose from amino acids derived from the proteins.

For example, the Inuit people can live in the Arctic for long periods of time on a diet that provides approximately 50% of their calories from fat. Their liver produces glucose from the amino acids in meat. In addition, they burn extensive amounts of acetyl coenzyme A, derived from fat, as fuel in their cells. Thus, nature has protected the Inuit who have little carbohydrate available to them in their diet. In short, carbohydrates are not an essential food for humans.

Most importantly, while we need carbohydrates, we do not need them in the volume that today's diets of three meals per day, plus snacks, often provide. And the main culprit in today's diets is carbohydrates from grains.

Diabetes specialists justify the intake of grain saying that glucose is an important nutrient. However, the body stores only a small amount (120 grams) of glucose as carbohydrate. Glucose molecules that cells don't take inside within four hours of absorption into the blood are converted to fatty acids for long-term storage in your fat cells, to be used for later energy production as needed. And given that the body also makes glucose from other foods we eat in addition to grain-based carbohydrates, the chances are that you are frequently overloading your body's capacity to utilize glucose. It does not matter the type of food the body acquires the glucose from — 120 grams are 120 grams!

Not all carbs are created equal

Since I am advising against the consumption of grain-based carbohydrates, you may wonder about plant-based carbohydrates, such as from fruits and vegetables, and how much of those I recommend. First, I do not recommend a specific quantity of carbohydrate, regardless of its source, to be consumed with any meal. This is because no carbohydrate has been found to be an essential nutrient for humans. Your liver can manufacture all the glucose the body needs from other nutrients such as amino acids even if your meal contains no carbohydrate. And since the liver can store only 120 grams of carbohydrate at a time, not much is needed if you are eating fruits and vegetables.

However, there are important differences among the types of plant-based carbohydrates that impact human health in different ways. It is helpful to understand this, because not all carbs are created equal. Different plant-based foods provide different amounts and types of carbs.

Plants with resistant starch

One class of carbohydrates is called "resistant starch," because their degradation products escape digestion in the small intestine of healthy individuals. This means they produce very little glucose that gets absorbed into the bloodstream. The content of naturally occurring resistant starch varies from one plant product to another, but overall, eating plants that contain resistant starch will have a lower impact on your blood sugar compared to the same volume of a grain-flour food. Examples of plant foods containing resistant starch are white beans, peas, banana flour from green bananas, raw slightly green bananas, lentils and specifically altered potatoes and corn.

Plants with low-glycemic carbs

The "glycemic index" is a number associated with a food's effect on the rise in a person's blood glucose level two hours after consumption of the food. Some foods produce carbohydrates that break down very slowly in digestion and therefore cause a gradual elevation in blood sugar. Other plant-based foods contain carbohydrates that are broken down faster and cause blood sugar to rise quickly. Many beans, lentils, nuts, and most vegetables are classified in the low glycemic index category. A few vegetables, such as carrots and potatoes, are higher in the glycemic index than vegetables like broccoli, cauliflower, asparagus, and other common dinner companions. Most fruits are low in their glycemic index compared to grains. The highest glycemic index plant-based foods are grains — wheat, oats, rice, barley — and foods made with those grains (pasta, pizza, noodles). This means that your blood sugar values measured two hours after a meal are likely to be significantly lower after a meal composed mainly of vegetables, compared to a meal containing grains or made from grain-flour products. See Appendix 1 for a comparison of how much carbohydrate is contained in various vegetables compared to grains.

Plants with oligosaccharides

While a molecule of grain flour can break down into thousands of molecules of glucose, an oligosaccharide typically contains only two to ten molecules of simple sugars. These sugars get attached to many amino acids and fat molecules and serve important biological functions in the body. Some of the oligosaccharides provide nourishment for health-promoting bacteria residing in the intestine. For babies, breast milk is a source of oligosaccharide to promote the growth of beneficial bacteria in their intestine. Jerusalem artichoke, burdock, chicory, leeks, onions, and asparagus are good sources of oligosaccharides.

Yacon, a tuber commonly cultivated in the Peruvian Andes, has a higher percentage of oligosaccharide compared to most other food items for humans. Some farmers in the US are trying to grow yacon and plants can be purchased from nurseries if you want to grow your own.

When you put all this together, the take-away is that the more plant-based foods you consume, except for grains, the better chances you have at keeping your blood sugar consistently low. This will help you avoid diabetes.

Natural sugars vs. glucose

Many people are confused about whether natural sugar, i.e., *sucrose,* is the same as glucose in your bloodstream. This form of sugar is found in fruit, berries, sugar cane, sugar beets, and other crops that can be boiled down into forms of sugar. The confusion is understandable because, when discussing diabetes, we always refer to the problem of having high blood "sugar." The same word "sugar" appears to be referring to the same item, so there is a tendency to think that eating any natural sugar increases your blood sugar.

But digesting natural sugar is not the same as filling your bloodstream with glucose. Sucrose contains equal parts of glucose and fructose. Both are absorbed as they're released in the intestine. But while the glucose adds to your blood sugar level almost immediately, fructose is absorbed only half as fast as glucose and must be further processed into glucose before it can elevate your blood sugar level.

This means eating a piece of fruit doesn't add the same amount of glucose to your bloodstream as quickly as eating an equal amount of carbohydrate as rice, mashed potatoes, or bread.

The same is true for milk sugar (*lactose*), which is made of 1 molecule of galactose and 1 molecule of glucose. Galactose must be further processed by the liver before it can elevate your blood sugar. The medical profession has done a poor job of educating people that natural sugar has not been shown to increase the incidence of complications in Type 2 diabetes. In fact, the medical profession may have unwittingly contributed to creating a prevailing culture in which people fear the natural sugars of whole fruit.

NATURAL SUGARS

Maltose   ● ● = 2 glucose

Sucrose   ● ★ = 1 glucose
                 1 fructose

Lactose   ● ◆ = 1 glucose
                 1 galactose

Most natural sugars are two linked-up single sugar molecules, as shown.

The human experience with natural sugar started when our hunter-gatherer ancestors experienced the sweetness of berries and fruits, possibly because the sweet taste indicated that the food was safe. Our personal experience with sweet taste starts as a baby when we consume lactose (milk sugar), or regular sugar. When any of these sugars come into contact with the sweet-sensing taste buds in the mouth, it sends signals to the brain which produces the sensation of sweetness.

Because there is some glucose in natural sugars, the brain causes the release of insulin from the pancreas. This triggers the transfer of glucose already in the blood into cells in the body to make room for the glucose expected to be absorbed from food in the gut. The elevation of blood sugar after digestion and absorption of the food then reassures the brain that glucose has been received as expected, a state of starvation has been averted, and fuel in the form of glucose is available for immediate or future use.

Through repetition of this experience, when any type of sugar stimulates the sweet-sensing taste buds, it produces a pleasing response because your brain has a learned experience of satisfaction based on nutritive value. Over time, the body associates the sweet taste with the imminent arrival of glucose in the blood. This is like receiving a paycheck. From experience, you know what it represents — soon to be available money in your bank account.

In short, eating a piece of fruit for breakfast or as a dessert does not deliver the same immediate glucose impact to your blood as eating a grain-based product such as toast, muffins, cake, or pie, so it is effectively healthier for you.

Usefulness of no-calorie sweeteners

Many people believe that using no-calorie sweeteners helps them reduce their intake of energy from natural sugars in food. However, there are many reasons why this is a misleading and counterproductive idea.

First, certain molecules of no-calorie sweeteners act through a separate receptor on the sweet-sensing taste buds on your tongue to send signals to the brain. These molecules do not contain any energy the body can use, but the brain generates the sensation of sweetness that could be interpreted as the entry of energy into the body, based on previous experience with the sweet sensation from natural sugars such as lactose, sucrose, and maltose. The brain, naturally, expects that there will soon be glucose to be absorbed, but when none enters the body, the brain can become confused and ultimately change its interpretation of the sensation of sweetness. This is like depositing your paycheck only to find out that the check does not represent money because the issuer's bank account did not have sufficient funds. After that experience, you begin attaching no importance to any future check you get from that issuer.

Worse, the brain's inability to accurately predict what should happen to your blood glucose levels after the sweet taste buds have been stimulated by artificial sweeteners could eventually cause it to misinterpret what you are eating when you consume real carbohydrates during a meal. This misinterpretation can then delay the satisfaction signal that occurs when the intensity of enjoyment is reduced — an important factor in your brain deciding to send the satiation signal as we discussed in the prior step. Based on the false assumption that you're not consuming energy when you use sweetness from a no-calorie sweetener to eat more of a carbohydrate preparation, your blood sugar can go higher than it would have otherwise.

Secondly, the prolonged use of a no-calorie sweetener could cause you to not fully appreciate the sensation of sweetness when you eat naturally sweet edibles such as fruits. To compensate, you might eventually begin adding no-calorie sweeteners to these, creating a spiraling "not sweet enough" syndrome. If you put two teaspoons of sugar in your mouth, the sweetness you experience is not double that of one teaspoon of sugar. This effect is just like how your other senses behave. For example, ten people singing the same note will not be perceived as being ten times louder than one person singing the note. In other words, loudness does not increase proportionately with the number of people singing. In the same way, once you become accustomed to the intensity of sweetness of a no-calorie sweetener, the taste of natural sugar in fruits may not be perceived as providing adequate sweetness because of the way your mechanism of taste perception works.

A third problem with no-sugar sweeteners is that they are often substituted for sugar in recipes for sweets such as desserts made with grain-flour. This leads people to believe it is okay to eat these foods since they contain no sugar. However, most desserts are also loaded with calories from butter, cream, nuts, and other ingredients. In this case, the purpose of eating sweets with no-calorie sweeteners and no added sugar to reduce energy intake is defeated by the presence of other energy nutrients.

Yet another problem is that the use of no-calorie sweetener can indirectly spur a craving to consume complex carbohydrates when your brain senses a significant lowering of blood sugar. In the past, the brain believed that it could expect glucose absorption soon after experiencing the sweet sensation. But the meaning of the sweet taste has been usurped. Your brain therefore may prompt you to eat a complex carbohydrate to make up for the missing glucose because the mouth-feel of complex carbohydrate and subsequent expectation of arrival of glucose in the blood remain intact. This can turn into a cycle of consuming no-calorie sweetened foods followed by a craving for real carbohydrates, which increases your risk of Type 2 diabetes.[7]

Avoid high sugar content drinks

There is a literal pandemic of beverages now produced with added sugar or high-fructose corn syrup, most of it in the form of soda and sweetened drinks. You may not realize the enormous amount of sugar in many of these drinks. While an eight-ounce glass of milk contains about three teaspoons of natural sugar, there are eight teaspoons of sugar in a can of regular soda.

I highly recommend weaning yourself off sodas and beverages with added sugar or high-fructose corn syrup to reduce your intake of carbohydrates.

Beer, wine, and spirits

Typically, beers, wines, and spirits contain between 3% and 40% ethanol (alcohol) by volume. The molecules of alcohol you consume are changed in the liver. The resulting chemicals may be inserted into the same metabolic line that uses glucose for your cellular energy production. This means that glucose molecules that would normally have been used for energy production remain unused, leaving them in the liver or bloodstream.

In addition, beers and wines also contain sugars that contribute glucose. This explains why the body may convert almost all the excess glucose to fat to be stored in available areas — think beer belly — as well as contributing to high blood sugar.

When people drink alcohol, especially in a social setting, they also tend to munch on something that contains carbohydrates. This means that consuming alcohol can be a double whammy to your carb consumption if you are prediabetic or diabetic.

Eat a varied diet, not a "balanced" diet

The concept of eating any type of diet is different in this book, because I do not believe people can follow a strict diet with any degree of consistency. Other than reducing your grain consumption as much as possible, I offer you no other specific rules to follow as to what to eat.

In my view, the more varied your diet, the better chances you have of supplying your body with the full range of nutrients humans need, including glucose, amino acids, fatty acids, vitamins, and minerals. Each cell in the body requires multiple nutrients to survive, sustain its internal functions, and create products such as enzymes, hormones, and proteins. It is not the presence of a single nutrient that produces the unique biological effect of a cell, but a specific mix of nutrients in the fluid around each cell and the readiness of the cell to respond. What is thus needed is a varied diet that supplies the varied nutrient needs of the body.

So if you have a tendency to eat the same foods over and over, I suggest you need to branch out and try new fruits, vegetables, spices, and meats. Vary your menu using the most seasonally available, freshest items because fresh foods eaten in season still contain most of their nutrients. Try new recipes where ingredients are mixed differently to create various combinations of nutrients in the food you consume. Think of eating as a chance to explore the great diversity of nutrients available to humankind.

Unfortunately, nutritional science today has become hung up on the concept of eating a "balanced diet." As currently understood, a balanced diet is based on eating a variety of foods within and among the "five food groups" to derive all the nutrients your body needs. You are advised to balance each type of food, choosing, for example, foods that are low in fat if you have already consumed something high in fat. You are supposed to moderate your portion sizes so that you can enjoy all the foods you like while controlling the intake of calories and total amount of fat, saturated fat, cholesterol, sugars, and sodium. The serving amounts are determined based on the average content of nutrients in foods and average daily utilization of the same nutrients in the body adjusted for age, gender, and activity level, starting from age two years and up.

The problem with this view of a balanced diet is that the nutrient amount currently recommended for intake during each day and each meal is a calculated average based on scientific studies of the actual amounts people consume over a period of time. Although it can be helpful to have some type of recommendation based on averages from different studies, it is just a rough approximation. The actual amount of nutrients that most people consume during meals is usually vastly different.

Furthermore, averages are not very reliable. The accuracy of averages in research on nutrients depends on how well the study conditions were controlled, whether the study subjects had the nutrient under study in their system already, and, if so, at what level, and the concentration of the nutrient in the food consumed. In my view, applying a recommendation to any specific individual is suspect because people do not live in controlled environments.

My belief is, your nutritional requirements depend completely on your individual situation, which changes day by day. One day you may have a busy 16-hour schedule, full of activity and stress. Following that, your body may be severely deficient in certain nutrients needed to produce more stress hormones. Another day, you may do intensive physical exercise and your body becomes deficient in the minerals and vitamins used to produce muscle energy.

Take into account these differing circumstances in your daily life. It is almost impossible to suggest a balanced diet based on average daily use under these conditions.

EAT AND ENJOY
WITH NO DIABETES

THIS STEP is aimed at helping you keep your blood sugar down after you lower it using the seven steps described above.

But, first, let us review some basics of how the body uses food to survive.

Nourishing your cells

The human body contains trillions of independent living cells, grouped into different functional units, with the brain acting as the control center. The brain receives information on a regular basis from specific organs and systems in the body regarding nutrient deficiencies and creates the sensation of hunger when the cumulative nutrient need reaches a threshold level. The relative strength of a nutrient's contribution to the hunger signal increases corresponding to the degree of deprivation of that nutrient reported to the brain.

After a meal, the digested nutrients are absorbed into the blood circulation and are pumped by the heart into the aorta, the blood vessel that divides and divides into smaller and smaller tubes called arteries, arterioles, and finally capillaries. The fluid part of the blood (but not the blood cells) leaks out through small holes in the capillary walls, ferrying nutrients to each cell. About 200 varieties of cells in the body take in different nutrients according to what is needed for their assigned functions, in addition to those needed for routine upkeep and maintenance. This clarifies the need for eating a variety of foods in a timely fashion as prompted by the sensation of hunger.

Similar to the control center in the brain, each cell nucleus regulates the entry of each and every nutrient into a cell. However, unlike the unlimited entry of nutrients into the body, the cell nucleus is stricter in limiting nutrient entry to only those needed at the time. The nucleus receives information regarding deficiencies of nutrients needed by different working groups inside the cell, called organelles.

As mentioned, the nutrient needs of each cell is predicated on its work assignment. For example, calcium is needed by bone cells, iron by red blood cells, iodine by thyroid cells, etc. For every nutrient needed by a cell, there are receptors on the cell wall to which nutrients get attached. The attachment results in the transmission of signals to the nucleus regarding the availability of that nutrient. Only if there is a need does the nucleus instruct opening the channel through which the nutrient can now enter the cell. In other words, the entry of a nutrient into a cell is based strictly on need, regardless of its availability. Without this control, the cell would be saturated with whatever nutrients are in excess in the surrounding fluid.

In a person with diabetes, glucose molecules are present in abundance outside each cell in the body. As you have learned though, the nucleus is informed of the presence of glucose by the attachment of insulin to its receptor on the cell wall. However, if the cell does not need additional fuel, because it is already producing sufficient energy from fatty acids, the nucleus will not cause the channel designed for entry of glucose into the cell to open.

Endocrinologists explain this as evidence of cellular resistance to insulin, without clarifying how can organs such as muscles keep producing energy and work while refusing entry of glucose. This is similar to a dinner guest who is full refusing to eat more food put on the plate, while the host complains that the guest is resisting feeding. However, as you learned, my explanation is that the cell simply does not need glucose, as it is functioning perfectly well with fatty acids as its fuel.

Reactivating your natural system of eating and enjoyment

Given the above description of how the body uses nutrients, in this step, I will explain how you can return to eating in the manner that nature intended humans (and all animals) to use food. Nature programmed the control center in the brain of all babies to be able to consume food to fulfil our nutrient needs right down to the cellular level. Without this system, we would not survive. You practiced this way of eating as an infant and a toddler.

The same faculties of eating regulation and control are still in your brain, and you can reactivate them. The fact is, the right cure for Type 2 diabetes is to return to listening to your natural regulatory mechanism of eating for nutrition. How to accomplish this is the main focus of this step.

———

Proof that the brain knows how you should eat

The best way to think about how you can relearn to eat to avoid or reverse Type 2 diabetes is what I call "eating like a toddler." Let me explain why there is proof that this makes sense.

When hungry, babies of all types — birds, animals, and humans — eat foods they enjoy (i.e., that taste good) to obtain the nutrients needed for normal growth and development. The brain, using the pleasurable feelings of enjoyment as a controlling mechanism, initiates the hunger signal when enough nutrient resupply is needed and signals that the act of eating can terminate by reducing the intensity of enjoyment. In other words, babies stop eating when the food is not as enjoyable relative to what it was when they started eating.

Is there any proof that the brain knows that you need specific nutrients and directs you to eat them? Is there any evidence to suggest that humans have a sophisticated mechanism to select from among various natural foods and consume enough quantities to meet the nutrient needs of a growing, active, and changing body?

The answer is yes. The evidence comes from an experiment conducted in the US that took place over 70 years ago. The experiment used infants newly weaned from breast milk and gave them a wide selection of foods to choose from on their own, without any adult prompting or assistance. In this experiment, it was demonstrated that each infant naturally chose an assortment of foods that provided all the nutrients their body needed to remain healthy and growing. (See Appendix 2 for a full accounting of the experiment).

While we might be tempted to think that infants would choose the same food over and over, or might veer towards only sweet or salty foods, or might not eat enough or too much, this experiment proved that *babies appear to choose their foods according to their nutrient needs, not just taste preference.* The experiment seems to verify that the brain truly has a mechanism to monitor the nutrient levels in the body, assess what new ones are required, and stop food intake as nutritional needs are met.

If you accept that this experiment is evidence of how the brain monitors and regulates the intake of nutrients in infants, it is only logical to conclude that this regulatory mechanism exists in adults. There is no evidence to suggest that any of our natural regulatory mechanisms in the body are lost as we grow into adulthood. For example, our body's mechanism to regulate our water intake through our sense of thirst does not appear to disappear as we grow from infancy to adulthood. Our mechanism to regulate breathing remains the same between infancy and adulthood, based on the concentration of oxygen in the blood, the need to exhale carbon dioxide, and the need to maintain proper acidity of the blood.

It thus seems clear that when the adult brain knows we are lacking in nutrients, it prompts us with the same clear message as it did when we were children: "I'm hungry, and this is what I need to eat."

Returning to the "toddler" way of eating

In essence, what I am suggesting is that you return to this "toddler" way of eating, which is based on both the brain's signaling of the need for nutrients as well as the enjoyment of food. As a toddler, you knew when you were truly hungry and that when you ate, you experienced the pleasure of eating. As a toddler, you likely ate slowly, chewed the food, and could not be hurried, even when parents encouraged you to speed up the process. How much you ate as a toddler was based on your own satisfaction, despite any enticements or threats from parents or caregivers to "eat everything on your plate."

Today, the toddler way of regulating food intake and meal enjoyment is also the natural way for adults to reverse Type 2 diabetes. Of course, you will be right to say that being an adult is not the same as being a toddler; you have responsibilities to others, need to earn a living, have family obligations, experience mental and emotional challenges, and so on.

However, I invite you to remember: you were once a toddler, a vibrant learning being. Although you now exist in a universe created in your mind based on your own experiences as you grew up into an adult, your natural mental and emotional capabilities, especially those related to your food intake and enjoyment, are still very similar in structure and function to your toddler years. They are all amenable to reactivation.

Let me tell you how you can revert to eating like a toddler, paying attention to your hunger and satiation signals, and not overeating out of stress, emotional need, or other reasons that ultimately cause you to gain weight and raise your blood sugar.

Eat slowly and consciously!

This advice may sound old-fashioned, but it is truly the foundation of relearning to eat for health. Choosing the right foods and appreciating the nutrition in them are analogous to appreciating the colors and shapes that make a painting visually appealing. Feeling the mix of nutrients in your mouth is like listening closely to sound waves of a symphony (rock music song) with their different duration, speed, and grouping that hit your eardrum in an orderly sequence and make the music pleasing.

Nutrients are the elements that trigger the wonderful signals used by your brain to create your sense of enjoyment during a meal. Nutrients enter your mouth as a mixture of unpredictable variety and concentration in each item of food. Eating slowly allows more time for their signals to reach your brain. In short, each meal should be an anticipated, pleasurable event. Starting a meal in response to hunger sensation, rather than scarfing down food out of stress, is the best way to make sure of that.

Since no one else but you can know your body's immediate nutrient needs, as they depend on your activities and your prior eating, you must rely on your own internal monitoring and metering mechanisms to ensure you consume an adequate amount of nutrients during a meal. Your ability to assess the nutrition in your food is directly proportional to the amount of time nutrients remain in contact with your taste and smell receptors. The more time you keep nutrients in contact with them, the more signals your brain receives — and the more enjoyment of food you will have.

You will be amazed as you pass age 40 how little food you need during any given meal to sustain yourself until the next meal, unless your job requires strenuous physical activity. But while you need less food, you still require the same quality and diversity of nutrients as you did when you were younger. In short, reducing the quantity of food you consume need not translate into reduced pleasure of eating.

Your mission during a meal should be to eat what you enjoy and, more importantly, to enjoy what you eat.

The primary objective of this advice is to help you learn to stop eating any item of food when your body does not need the actual nutrition from it. You can ascertain this by listening closely to your brain's hunger and satisfaction signals. Ask yourself when you are tempted to eat something, "Am I eating because I am hungry? Or am I eating for some other reasons?"

Then, after you begin eating, assess when you no longer need to eat any remaining food on your plate by paying attention to the diminished intensity of your pleasure in eating.

These natural control mechanisms will help you change your past learned behaviors to eat until you feel your stomach full. You will begin to empty your fat cells, lose weight, and begin living a healthy, diabetes-free life.

Let me make an analogy for eating consciously and slowly. Imagine yourself among a group of people scattered inside a closed 10 X 10 foot room. Someone releases a fragrance into the room from a concealed canister. Within seconds, you know the nature and concentration of the fragrance regardless of your location in the room. A few molecules of the perfume extracted from the air you breathe in are enough for your brain to know the properties of the perfume.

Similarly, the sensing of only several molecules with your taste and smell receptors is all that is needed for your brain to understand the nutrients being swallowed. Put another way, there is no reason to swallow a lot of food without really enjoying it. The antidote to this is to become a conscious eater, enjoying more of what you eat while reducing the intake of food that is not enjoyed.

Reflect on why you developed fast eating patterns and change them!

If you reflect on your life, I'm sure you will admit that most of the time, you don't eat slowly. In our fast-paced lives, we tend to eat very quickly. Working people often gulp down their breakfast and lunch, some while driving or sitting at their desk at work. Even family dinner times may be hectic as parents are pressured to get the meal on the table after returning home from work so the children can have time to do homework or other activities. In my experience, most people don't spend sufficient time to truly savor their food, chew slowly, and pay attention to their body's signals.

Eating fast is not a natural human way to eat. If you look at infants sucking on the breast or at a bottle, they usually go slowly, starting and stopping several times during a feeding. The physical contact with the mother and the availability of milk reassure and please the baby. When infants are introduced to solid food, they begin sensing the various flavors and tastes on their taste buds and smell receptors. They start establishing their food preferences.

Eating habits, attitudes, and unconscious feelings about foods are created at this stage of life. Of course, these early habits are later influenced by one's family and national cultures, as food choices and flavors are passed from generation to generation, strengthened by association with rituals and the eating habits of your country. But no matter what culture they grow up in, most children still eat slowly. The classic admonition from parents around the world is telling their child to, "Hurry up and finish your food."

For adults, the changeover to eating fast occurs for different reasons at different times. You may have started rushing through meals during your childhood years so that you could run outside to play with friends. Or you may have started eating fast in high school or college so that you could do homework or spend time on the phone or computer with a boyfriend or girlfriend, or just to go to your room to avoid your parents. Or it might have begun as an adult when you started working in a real job and found yourself under pressure to devote your lunch hour (or just 30 minutes for many people) to work rather than to enjoying your food.

Little by little, most adults begin adapting to eating fast all the time, paying less and less attention to their choice of food and their body's reactions to it. They cave in to work schedules that allow little time to eat. Lack of time and the pressure to get things done often force them to take larger bites in order to quickly finish a meal. The same factors also cause them to speed up the rate of chewing and to swallow it quickly, what we often call "gobbling down" food. With busy families, many adults often eat lunch or dinner alone with little opportunity to "dine" and enjoy a slow meal while talking. Fast-food restaurants become part of many adults' weekly routine — and the term "fast" applies not only to how quickly they receive their food but how speedily they consume it.

Another consequence of eating fast is that it changes your sensitivity to your body's signals to stop eating. In your younger days, you were apt to respond more often to the sensory signals coming from your mouth. When your brain decided that you had gotten enough nutrients from consuming an item of food to meet the needs of your body, you responded by stopping eating that food.

But as you got older, though, you may have started using signals other than those coming from your mouth to terminate the act of eating. If you frequently ate food without enjoying it and without paying attention to it, you began to lose touch with knowing when to stop. Over time, you trained your brain to prompt you to stop eating only when you finally felt your stomach being very full, if not bloated. This increasingly became an automatic response during mealtime for you, even though you may have known full well that you were eating too much.

All these habits have reorganized your brain's former connections about food and established new ones that reinforce efficiency, speed, and the practicality of eating over the enjoyment of food and the pleasure of nourishing your body. Today, whenever you eat too fast to really enjoy what you are eating, whenever you clean your plate just to finish your meal (or get to the dessert faster), and whenever you indulge in food without being hungry, you continue to reinforce these neural connections and transform them into the only pathway that comes into your brain from eating.

As a result, you become increasingly unaware of the high levels of carbohydrate, fat, salt, and sugar content of the foods you are consuming because you simply are not taking the time to taste them.

Lessons in how to eat slowly

The act of eating slowly consists of three different stages:

- First, you experience the qualities of the food in your mouth by taking the time to chew it.
- Second, you decide whether the food is still appealing to you — before, during, and after chewing.
- Third, you swallow the food.

Repeat this process with each bite until you sense that the food no longer gives you the same enjoyment as when you started. Then you are done with your meal.

The best way to train yourself in this new way of eating is to focus on your chewing. The more aware you are of the jaw and mouth motions involved in chewing, the more you'll fully experience and enjoy the food before it disappears down your throat. You should be deliberate in chewing, feeling the force of each chewing motion. This will allow you to concentrate on the sensations generated during chewing.

Your goal is to literally taste and enjoy every bite of food as it sits in your mouth. When you chew it with the conscious intention of experiencing its nutrients on your taste and smell receptors, it completely changes the experience of eating, versus simply biting into food, smashing it for a second or two with your teeth, then swallowing it. Chewing slowly fully breaks up the food, creating new surfaces from which flavor-producing nutrients can be liberated. Proteins in general and meats in particular require more chewing compared to carbohydrates and cooked vegetables.

Enzymes that are secreted by the salivary gland aid this process. Some food is mixed with an enzyme called *ptyalin*, which breaks up the complex carbohydrates, releasing the sugar called maltose. Sweet-sensing receptors on the tongue cannot detect the complex carbohydrates themselves, only the maltose released in chewing. Less than 5 percent of all the complex carbohydrates that are eaten will be affected by ptyalin. However, enough maltose can be released in the oral cavity for it to register with your sweet-sensing taste receptors and that is what your brain enjoys.

Another enzyme, called *lipase,* breaks up fat, releasing its molecules. Agitation and warming of the food during chewing allows fat-associated nutrients to waft up the back of the throat where they stimulate the smell receptors, which need to detect only several of the molecules in each bite to register the odors and create enjoyment. If you savor cooked or barbecued chicken, beef, or fish by chewing it slowly, you will notice that your nose becomes increasingly sensitive to the odors, contributing to your pleasure of eating these foods.

Appreciating the combination of sensations from the textures, temperature, and flavor or "heat" from spices, and the smell signals in your nose creates the full experience of each bite of food during a meal. Reliance on your taste and smell receptors to enjoy the quality and to determine the quantity of food consumed shows that you are in charge of your body.

Your sense of enjoying each bite of food is the result of the unique construct of your brain's processing system. The brain compares what it was expecting when it created the sensation of hunger versus the signals generated by your taste and smell receptors. This experience changes in intensity as the meal progresses, usually rising in enjoyment at first, then descending. The experience can differ from one meal to the next, based on the differing foods you are eating and the incoming nutrients in them. But overall, this progression from great enjoyment to lesser enjoyment is what you want to look for.

Swallowing food without enjoying the flavor of it is like flushing a delicious dish down the drain without tasting it. Only when food is properly chewed can you receive and understand the full palette of its tastes, flavors, and sensations.

Additional tips to keep in mind

Each time you eat, you have the opportunity to embed this new way of eating in your brain. The key to establishing a new eating behavior is to change each and every element that defines your past processes of eating. You can force your brain to concentrate on your new behavior by replacing as many of the practices that remind you of your old eating pattern with new ones, such as these:

- When you take small bites, you can better understand even the smallest amount of food you consume. Therefore, adjust the bite size of your food. If you are taking large bites such that you need to "park" the food in your cheek while you chew part of it, you have taken too big a bite.

- Always put food on your tongue when you introduce it into your mouth. Feel the texture of the food before you start chewing. This lets you enjoy the food from the moment you put it in your mouth, as enjoyment starts with awareness.

- During the meal, use your tongue to rotate the food around your mouth. This churning releases more taste and flavor-producing nutrients. To register the released nutrients with taste sensors, you should bring the chewed portion of the food back on the tongue. Depending on the texture, you may need to switch the rest of the food to the other side and repeat chewing and tasting until you have fully enjoyed each bite of food. If you swallow before enjoying your food, you're defeating the purpose of eating.

- Separate out the various elements of the food to understand them individually. You know from experience that you can enjoy food cut as paper thin as a slice of carrot, cucumber, or single potato chip in your mouth. When you put a stack of any of these in your mouth, your taste buds will not come in contact with each individual slice, and you will enjoy it less.

- Change what you drink to accompany the meal to increase your conscious awareness that you are developing new habits of eating. Drink water instead of your usual drink with the meal. If you are already drinking water with your meal, try a different type, like filtered, carbonated, bottled, or drink warm water rather than cold.

- If you are eating spicy foods, have thin slices of fresh vegetables such as cucumber, carrot, turnip, radish, jicama, etc., available to nibble on between bites. Water from these will clean your taste buds while you get a chance to understand the natural flavor of each one.

- If you have a favorite chair or place you sit to eat your meal, change it.

- Try new recipes instead of making the same ones over and over. My newest book, *The Diabetes-Free Cookbook and Exercise Guide,* can introduce you to more than 80 new recipes.
- Use new utensils and a new plate.
- Buy smaller portions of meat and fish.
- As much as possible, serve yourself the type and quantity of each item of food you want to eat rather than letting someone else serve you. This is to prevent the temptation of eating all that's served in order to avoid wasting food or to please the host. When in doubt, serve small quantities.

Eat like Europeans

If you have ever travelled in Europe, you may have seen how the French, Italians, Spanish, Germans, and Scandinavians all take time for big lunches (their main meal of the day). Whether they eat in a café, restaurant, or at home, they take a full hour to have lunch, eating slowly, forkful by forkful, while truly savoring the food. Compared to fast eaters, most Europeans seem to take forever to finish their plate, even though the portions are usually smaller than what Americans typically serve. Think of your next lunch or dinner as being a delectable dining event in Italy or France.

Give the act of eating your respect and undivided attention

Eating consciously is about focusing your attention only on the meal. When people are thinking of other things or watching TV, it forces the conscious part of the brain to take over, and eating becomes an unconscious task.

Magnetic resonance imaging (MRI) studies of brain activity show that when people try to concentrate simultaneously on two demanding tasks, total brain activity decreases rather than doubling. This could be because the conscious brain concentrates on the one activity (e.g., work or TV) while delegating the second one (eating) to the subconscious brain. While your brain is capable of multitasking, such multitasking does not produce optimal performance. For example, if you pay attention to the TV or a work conversation while eating, the chewing and tasting are handed off to the subconscious part of your brain, which should have been processing the signals coming from the taste and smell receptors in your mouth. Meanwhile, the conscious mind is distracted and cannot make the best choices about your food consumption.

The evidence for this is solid. Increased food consumption while watching television has been identified as one of the key contributors to obesity. When you watch TV, your brain receives thousands of messages every second. Out of the multiple signals from the mouth, eyes, and ears received by the brain during a meal while watching television, the brain is forced to select one to pay primary attention to, meanwhile scanning the rest of the information for other messages that could be valuable. As the images change on the TV, your brain is constantly shifting its orientation from the signals coming from the mouth to the rapidly changing sights and sounds on the screen.

Out of all sensory input into your brain, you are programmed to receive messages most strongly through your eyes. If the mind pays no attention when you taste food, it is as if you have not tasted it and the quantity of food consumed is determined by your subconscious mind, as just explained. With repeated episodes of eating combined with attention-grabbing distractions, overeating becomes a normal behavior. No matter how much you concentrate during your meal, other things such as reading, listening intensely to a conversation, and watching an event make it difficult to regulate your intake based on sensory signals. The importance of this cannot be underestimated. Try to eat your meals in a calm, peaceful environment without distraction so that you can consciously focus on what you eat, how it tastes, and how much you are consuming.

The importance of noticing the intensity of your enjoyment

If eating is about taking in nutrients for the survival of the body, stopping consumption should reflect when your body has received enough of the nutrients it needs. This takes time, however, given that an ordinary meal consists of multiple food groups, each containing a mixture of nutrients. This means that an accurate assessment of the composition and concentration of the nutrients consumed is not fully known to the brain until after the food is completely digested and absorbed, a process that can take hours. This is why the body supplies other signals that it is time to stop eating.

As you learned earlier, the most important one of these signals is the change in the pleasantness of the food in your mouth. This is your clue to stop eating regardless of how much is left on the plate or the availability of more in the kitchen.

Moreover, to understand the drop in the intensity of pleasure related to the food you're eating, you must be aware of the pleasure of eating that food. This is how conscious eating helps you. Only when you pay attention to the food inside your mouth are you able to sense the reduction in enjoyment of that food. Multitasking and distractions during your meal keep your brain from noticing the transition from enjoyment to lack of enjoyment in what you're eating.

I cannot give you advice about how to rank your enjoyment of food in a way that can be measured. As yet, no system exists to help humans accurately quantify and express their enjoyment of eating in absolute numbers, like measuring the "heat" in different chili peppers or the temperature of rare vs. well-done meat. You need to rely on your own senses to learn when food ceases to be enjoyable to you as you eat a meal.

The fact that almost every bite of food you eat has multiple nutrients, each stimulating the taste and smell receptors at different strengths, makes it hard to notice when the intensity of your enjoyment changes. Perhaps the best scale you can use to assess the intensity of your enjoyment of eating is to compare each consecutive bite to the very first one you took. Unless you pay close attention, you will miss the diminishing intensity of enjoyment over the continuous stimulus of a meal, just as you would when listening to music and trying to read at the same time.

If you aren't sure whether you might be sensing a lower enjoyment of your food, take a sip of water after food is swallowed to give your brain time to assess the situation, especially after eating complex carbohydrates. Warm water cleanses the taste buds better than cold water. When taste buds are already occupied with nutrients, they can't accept freshly released nutrients in the next bite of food. Washing the taste buds with water unclogs the taste pores to accept new molecules. If drinking so much is not amenable to you, just sip water every couple of minutes during the meal. The objective is not to fill your stomach with water but to cleanse your taste buds so you can assess whether the food's taste is still enjoyable.

Note that drinking water does not remove the molecules that occupy the smell sensors in your nose. But if you breathe out through your nose, the air current will dislodge the nutrient molecules and carry them out. Another choice is to sip a warm drink such as hot tea, as the vapors from it can create the movement of warm air up through the nose, facilitating the removal of molecules in the smell receptors.

Sipping wine also facilitates cleaning the smell receptors because of the alcohol vapors. It is not known, however, whether alcohol in the wine cleans the taste receptors as well. It's possible that those who savor wine and try to make distinctions between which grapes it was made from and its unique aromas and flavors are also simply paying more attention to the food they eat. By concentrating on changes in flavor due to the presence of acidity, fruitiness, and tannin in each wine, wine connoisseurs become even more conscious of the smallest differences in the taste of their food. If the wine is "paired" with the food (meaning it is chosen to compliment the flavors of the food), many people become even more aware of the harmonies among the tastes and smells in their mouth.

Developing your sense of taste to be increasingly precise is possible because the processing structures in the neurons of your brain are capable of processing signals with very minimal difference. Most people can easily taste the difference between a peach and an apricot, a pear and an apple, and Mahi-mahi and tilapia. But you also can, with practice, train yourself to detect the minute differences between plums and pluots, Fuji and Gala apples, and brown trout and rainbow trout. Try it and you will be surprised at what your taste and smell receptors are capable of.

The brain also assigns different sets of neurons to process information based on priorities assigned to specific groups of signals. When you pay close attention to your food, the brain makes specific changes in the connecting pathways based on detailed differences in signals and priorities. In fact, it has been shown that when you pay attention to any task you're doing, the brain releases nerve growth agents that consolidate the connections between neurons, helping to wire them together for future coordinated action. In addition, nerve cells produce a number of proteins that allow information to be stored. This helps you remember the experience. This capability of the brain is very useful for establishing a new way of eating based on having an increasingly sophisticated palette.

What to do about "lingering hunger"

As you transition into conscious and slow eating, you may feel that your hunger does not abate at the end of each meal even as you pay attention to the signals of satisfaction we've been discussing. One reason for this, confirmed by studies, is that during meals, most people can detect a reduction in the intensity of taste of a flavor more than they can detect the drop in intensity of their hunger. In other words, sometimes your hunger may not fully subside during a particular meal, although you no longer enjoy the taste of it. If you feel this, the solution is to tap into your willpower to stop eating when you sense the lack of enjoyment even if you are still hungry. Your brain knows that your hunger will be satisfied in the course of the next meals.

This brain training is similar to other repetitive activities in your life. Consider reading a very long book. You can read a little at a time, knowing that you can come back to it in the next sitting. Your brain does not experience any lack of enjoyment from reading in spurts. What you accomplish in subsequent readings is simply added onto the pages you read until you finish the book.

Eating is the same. You may not consume all the nutrients you need during just one meal, but you can assure yourself that there will be other meals to come. Also, the body is constantly changing in its needs. This is why even when you feel satisfied with one type of food on your plate, other foods not yet eaten can still seem appealing because they have other nutrients needed by the body. Once your brain can be assured of the fact that you'll have opportunities to eat again, you'll be able to stop eating before you feel full. Slowly, this new way of eating will become natural, and it will take less and less willpower to stop before you get to the point of overeating.

If you did not obtain all the nutrients you needed in a meal, the brain knows it can correct any unmet needs in subsequent meals. As long as there are adequate nutrient reserves in the body, the brain can wait several hours for complete absorption of nutrients from one meal before reassessing what else you need — and regenerating the sensation of hunger again.

This confirms why humans rely on multiple meals of varying sizes to get all their needed nutrients on any given day. In many ways, it is not so different from what you may already do. When you eat a small breakfast, you may already tell yourself that it is enough as lunch will soon follow. Similarly, if you eat a large breakfast, you can be okay with just a small lunch, knowing that dinner will fill in your hunger gap.

In short, your brain's nutrition monitoring system detects not only what the body absorbed during a meal but also what was not acquired. If you can begin to apply this same thinking to all your meals, you will soon train yourself to be satisfied with a smaller volume of food at each meal, knowing that you will consume more nutrition at a later meal.

EPILOGUE

T O LOWER and maintain your blood sugar within normal limits, and ultimately reverse your diabetes (and possibly lose weight, too), you need to create new habits that reinforce your goal to regulate your food intake. Here is a summary checklist of the things you have learned in this book:

- Significantly reduce grain and grain-based foods as much as possible. Grains are the culprits that trigger the "fatty acid burn switch" which forces your body to change from burning glucose to burning fatty acids on a regular basis. This switch leaves glucose in your bloodstream, which is the cause of high blood sugar and eventually diabetes.
- Any time you think of food, remember that the body is looking for nutrients, because the mouth has no separate receptors to identify food groups such as carbohydrates, proteins, or fat. And you have no clear idea of what nutrients are lacking in the body when you feel the desire to eat.
- Let your subconscious mind help you to select food based on your internal need for specific nutrients and the potential availability of the nutrients in the food items presented to you at that time.
- Limit your food items to those that require chewing before swallowing. This will help ensure that the nutritional molecules of food register in your mouth and contribute to your

enjoyment of the food, which will help you know when to stop eating.

- Every time you think of eating, remind yourself to eat slowly and savor your food. Form a mental picture of each chewing motion and of enjoying the taste. Slow down the speed of chewing from what you have done in the past and chew each bite of food thoroughly to release and enjoy the nutrients. Each time you do this, your brain connections change. If you can learn to imagine terminating a meal based on the loss of taste satisfaction, you can more easily do it for real during a meal.

- Pay attention to the sensory mechanisms in your body that allow you to respond to its natural signals of hunger and satisfaction. Following these will allow you to consume food with only occasional intake in excess of your immediate nutritional needs.

- Consume all liquids except water by sipping. This will ensure more registration of dissolved nutrients.

- When you eat out, try a new restaurant or order a new entrée. When you travel or go on a vacation, look forward to enjoying as much of your eating experience as possible. However, you need to bring the same mindset to each meal, always remembering you have more time to enjoy each bite of food.

Healthy living, diabetes free

Whatever your current age, the recommendations in this book will help you age more happily. When you achieve your goal of maintaining normal blood sugar, you will find yourself having more energy, feeling better about yourself, and finally enjoying one of the most meaningful activities of life — eating. Each meal will become a true sensory experience that delights you and, at the same time, reinforces your ability to eat for nourishment. Realizing that without putting glucose-producing foods in your mouth, your blood sugar can't go up, and you will avoid consuming food items that lead to high blood sugar and diabetes.

The most significant challenge for you as an adult is to achieve a mental framework of relaxed enjoyment during mealtimes. Of course, as an adult, you have probably become conditioned to eat a certain volume of food based on the time of day and location of the meal, such as a cafeteria, restaurant, or home, or the occasion, such as sporting events, movies, formal celebrations, or outdoor gatherings. However, you now know that it is possible to retrain your brain and become conscious of your eating behaviors.

Knowing the natural mechanism that underlies the hunger instinct should give you the confidence to strive for new habits. It will take time, but you can overcome the challenges, mostly external, and learn the skills to reverse your Type 2 diabetes. You can develop the smarts to become immune to image marketing and cultivate a lifestyle in which you eat what you enjoy, enjoy what you eat, and eat less of what you can't enjoy.

As you learn to maintain normal blood sugar by practicing conscious eating at every meal, you will find yourself automatically eating better and healthier, while enjoying it more. You will chew your food with great appreciation for its nutrients. You will taste more of its flavors, spices, textures, and unique qualities from each component of a recipe. You will be paying attention to what your brain tells you about your hunger and satisfaction. You will become more conscious of what to eat and how much of it, and you will reconnect with your body's natural rhythms for eating and activity.

Make the needed changes one at a time. With each change, you will begin to establish new neural connections and create a pathway that makes your new eating behavior the automatic response. Each time you repeat the new way of eating, these connections are strengthened.

It can take weeks before you learn and master these new eating habits. It can take months of concentration and practice before the habits become automatic. However, as you become a veteran at it, you will improve listening closely to your brain and recognizing exactly what it tells you. This is possible because you have reset the goal of eating to meet the nutrient needs of your body, not to fill your belly. Your brain will direct what conscious and unconscious actions are needed to accomplish that objective during each meal. As you get good at this skill, you will gain more self-control to end your meal any time you want.

You will most likely need to exercise self-discipline to carry out this plan. It won't help if you quit before you start getting results. Remember that all these years, you practiced a certain way of consuming all the nutrients your body needed. It's only natural for your brain to resist learning other ways of accomplishing the same objective. This makes it harder for the new ways to compete with something at which you're already proficient. During the early stages of practicing this method, you'll catch yourself falling back to the old way of eating. This is because most of the pathways that were used for the old eating habit are still in the brain, available for the subconscious mind.

Also, one of the major reasons for sliding back to your old way of eating is consumption of foods that require practically no chewing.

The surest way to get back on track is deliberately selecting only foods with texture, paying attention to each chewing motion and enjoying the nutrients released in the mouth.

Use these moments of recognition as opportunities to remind yourself that your old way of eating was based on the belief that the more you ate, the more you enjoyed your food. This notion might have started in your infancy when your mother coaxed you to take one more bite to finish what was on the plate. A babysitter or day care worker may have reinforced this by telling your mother how good you were on that day because you ate well, and that message made your mother happy. A relationship between the quantity of food eaten and producing happiness could have been established from that time onwards.

Each time you catch yourself going back to the old way of eating, use the opportunity to feel satisfied that you were able at least to identify and correct that old eating habit. To establish the new way of eating, you must replace most of the signals produced in your mouth by the old way of eating with new ones. Otherwise, the brain will easily go back to the old way of eating as soon as it detects familiar signals coming from the mouth. For example, if many food items are ordinary to you, it's easy for the old way of eating to emerge without your awareness, unless you change to new food items just to help establish a new way of eating.

The most important time during the transition learning period is most likely your largest meal of the day, be it lunch or dinner. This means you need to be especially vigilant during this meal to eat slowly and consciously, savoring your food. Pay attention to the size of each bite; be aware of the feel of the food in the mouth; enjoy the flavors and the warmth or coldness of the food. Check your speed of chewing and the movement of the food inside your mouth and pay attention to when you stop chewing or swallow the chewed portion. If you do these actions wrong, you can trigger your old way of eating.

Reconnecting with your true body

Being in touch and in tune with your body is one of the keys to healthy aging. The more capable you are of self-regulating your food consumption, the better you will be at meeting your nutritional needs as you age, without gaining weight or weakening your body through disease, or risking maintaining your ongoing condition of Type 2 diabetes. As your energy expenditure changes over time, you will become better at sensing when your need for energy nutrients should be increased or reduced. You may grow old, but you will not grow fat or diabetic. You may slow down, but you will know how to feed your internal organs properly with the wide variety of nutrients they need to stay healthy and functioning. When you become deeply in touch with your body in the present moment, all your meals will become more satisfying and enjoyable.

Critical to firmly establishing this new lifestyle are the feelings of pride, self-esteem, and satisfaction you derive each time you do it right. Repeated positive feelings will establish in your memory that your new way of eating will help you preserve health and harmony among all the organs in your body.

Furthermore, after practicing this new way of eating for a while, you'll be able to catch yourself even before you start going down a wrong path, reverting to old ways. Once your new attitude towards eating is fully established, you'll only need to correct your way of eating occasionally because most of the time you'll be eating the right way.

As you become efficient in executing this plan, you will probably begin to feel your hunger better than in the past. Sometimes you'll feel hungry earlier in the day, especially if you have been physically or mentally active. Sometimes the reverse will happen — you simply won't feel hungry at the usual lunch or dinnertime.

This change in your hunger is proof that you are starting to listen to your internal regulatory system, which has been re-sensitized to your original toddler way of eating. Keep in mind that your new eating behavior is more natural, authentic, and in harmony with how humans evolved to eat for nutrition. This connection to your "humanness" will help you feel healthier, happier, and stronger. You will be less prone to fall victim to false or deceptive food advertising, to ineffective third-party diet programs, and to overeating to compensate for stress or problems in your life.

And most of all, you will have reversed your Type 2 diabetes and likely avoided the worst consequences of it as you age well into your future.

COMPARISON OF GRAINS AND OTHER SOURCES OF CARBOHYDRATES

IN CASE YOU doubt that grains are as bad for you as this book claims, look at the table below. The comparison of grains to many types of vegetables shows exactly how grains contain far more carbohydrate than any vegetable.

Remember: each 4 grams of carbohydrate is equal to 1 teaspoon of sugar. Eating a sandwich is like eating 6 teaspoons of sugar; a pizza is like 10 teaspoons of sugar; a cup of rice equals 12 teaspoons of sugar. Each time you eat grains, you are effectively filling your body with volumes of glucose that you probably cannot use immediately. Little by little, you fill your fat cells with unused glucose, converted into fatty acids and stored as fat. At some point, when fat is broken back into fatty acids, your muscles begin burning those rather than glucose, and excess glucose stays in the blood, thus high blood sugar and eventually diabetes.

The next time you reach for a sandwich, a bowl of rice, a slice of pizza, or a muffin, doughnut, or piece of pie, remind yourself that you are eating many teaspoons of sugar.

Comparison of Grains with Other Sources of Carbohydrates

Food item (approximate, as serving size may vary)	Grams of carbs
Bread, 2 slices	24
Breakfast cereal, 1 cup	30
12" sandwich roll (like a sub or hoagie) 1 roll	36
Pizza, 1 slice	40
Pasta, 2 ounces	40
Rice, 1 cup	48
Bagel, 1	48
English muffin	13
Alfalfa sprouts, raw, 100g	0.4
Artichoke Jerusalem, boiled, 100g	10.6
Asparagus, boiled, 100g	4
Bamboo shoots, canned, 100g	0.7
Bean sprouts, mung, raw, 100g	4
Beetroot, boiled, 100g	9.5
Broccoli, green, boiled, 100g	1.3
Broccoli, purple, boiled, 100g	1.3
Brussels sprouts, boiled, 100g	3.1
Cabbage, spring, boiled, 100g	0.6
Cabbage, Chinese, raw, 100g	1.4
Cabbage, red, raw, 100g	3.7
Cabbage, savoy, raw, 100g	3.9
Cabbage, white, raw, 100g	5
Capsicum pepper, green, raw 100g	2.6
Capsicum pepper, red, raw 100g	6.4
Carrots, young, raw, 100g	6
Cauliflower, boiled, 100g	2.3

Food item (approximate, as serving size may vary)	Grams of carbs
Celery, raw, 100g	0.9
Corn, baby sweetcorn, boiled, 100g	2.7
Corn kernels, canned, 100g	27
Corn-on-cob, boiled, plain, 100g	11.6
Curly kale, raw, 100g	1.4
Cucumber, unpeeled, raw 100g	1.5
Eggplant, raw, 100g	2.2
Endive (Escarole), 100g	2.8
Fennel, raw, 100g	1.8
Garlic, fresh, raw, 100g	16
Leeks, raw, 100g	2.9
Lettuce, cos, romaine, raw, 100g	1.7
Lettuce, iceberg, raw, 100g	1.9
Mushrooms, common, raw, 100g	3.4
Potatoes, new, boiled, 100g	18
Onions, raw, 100g	7.9
Parsnip, raw, 100g	12.5
Peas, frozen, raw, 100g	9.3
Peas, fresh, raw, 100g	11.3
Radish, red, raw, 100g	2
Spinach, raw, 100g	1.6
Squash, butternut, baked, 100g	7.4
Squash spaghetti, baked, 100g	18
Zucchini, raw, 100g	1.8
Sweet potato, baked, 100g	28
Tomatoes, canned, & liquid, 100g	3
Tomatoes, cherry, raw, 100g	3
Yam, baked, 100g	37.5

Comparison of nutrients from various grains vs. lentils, Brazil nuts, raisins, and mushrooms

A common claim is that whole grains contain many important nutrients. As the Table below shows, you can get nearly all the grain-associated nutrients from vegetables, nuts, fruits, and mushrooms. Use of spices and herbs will give you even more opportunities to get needed nutrients without having to consume the voluminous amount of glucose, of which thousands of molecules are present in each molecule of complex carbohydrate that constitute the bulk of a grain kernel.

100g portion	Wheat	Brown Rice	Corn	Lentils	Brazil nuts	Raisins	Mush-rooms
Fiber (g)	12.2	3.5	7.3	10.7	7.5	3.7	1
Calcium (mg)	29	23	7	56	160	50	18
Iron (mg)	3.2	1.4	2.7	6.5	2.4	1.9	0.4
Magnesium(mg)	126	143	127	47	376	32	9
Phosphorus(mg)	288	333	210	281	725	24	120
Potassium(mg)	363	223	287	677	659	749	448
Sodium (mg)	2	7	35	6	3	11	6
Zinc (mg)	2.6	2.0	2.2	3.3	4.0	0.2	1.1
Copper (mg)	0.4		0.3				0.5
Manganese(mg)	3.9	3.7	0.4			0.3	
Selenium (mg)	70.7		15.5		1917 (ug)		26 (ug)
Thiamin (mg)	0.4	0.4	0.3	0.8	0.6	0.1	0.1
Riboflavin (mg)	0.1	0.1	0.2	0.2		0.1	0.5
Niacin (mg)	5.4	5.0	3.6	2.6		0.8	3.8
Pantothenic acid (mg)	0.9	1.5	0.4	2.1		0.1	1.5
Vitamin B6 (mg)	0.3	0.5	0.6	0.5		0.1	0.1
Folate Total (ug)	38	20	19	479	22	5	25

SUMMARY OF EXPERIMENT ON INFANT EATING BEHAVIOR

BETWEEN World Wars I and II, Dr. Clara Davis conducted an experiment with 15 infants, aged six to eleven months.[8] Among them there were four infants who were underweight, suggesting that they had not been getting adequate nutrition. Five others had rickets, a medical condition due to inadequate intake of nutrients such as vitamin D and/or calcium. None of the babies had been given foods other than formula or milk before the study. This age was chosen because the children had no experience of adult foods and no preconceived prejudices or biases about them. The children remained in the program for six months to six years.

The children were presented with a selection of 34 different foods of both animal and vegetable origin. These items were known to contain all the necessary nutrients such as proteins, fats, carbohydrates, vitamins, and minerals that humans need for survival. The items were selected because they could generally be procured fresh year-round. The food items included only the following:

Water; grade A raw milk and cultured milk; table salt; uncooked apples, bananas, orange sections or strained orange juice; fresh pineapple either finely cut or ground; finely cut, peeled peaches; finely cut, peeled tomatoes; beets, turnips, cauliflower, lettuce, and spinach cut or ground; baked potatoes and bananas; cooked apples, carrots, peas, and cabbage cut or ground. Oatmeal (steel cut) and wheat (whole wheat ground and not heat-treated) were served raw. Oatmeal, corn meal (yellow), and barley (whole grains) were cooked in a double boiler for three hours. To prepare the grains, one cup of cereal was cooked in five cups of water. Ry-Krisp made of whole rye flour and water with one percent common salt added was offered. The meats were lean beef and loin lamb chop from which 50% of the fat was removed before grinding and broiling without water loss. Cooked bone marrow was also offered, as was bone jelly made by boiling four pounds of veal bones in three quarts of water until one quart remained.

Chicken, sweet breads, brains, liver, and kidneys were finely cut and cooked in covered casseroles in a steamer. Fish (haddock) finely cut or ground, cooked in a covered casserole in a steamer was also offered, as were eggs served raw and soft poached.

All foods were prepared as simply as possible, unmixed and unaltered except in some cases by cooking in the simplest manner. Some foods were served both raw and cooked. Cooking was done without the loss of soluble substances and without the addition of salt or seasonings. Each food, including salt, milk, and water was served in a separate dish on a tray.

The infants were free to eat with their fingers or in any way they could. If an infant consumed an entire portion of an item, the size of the portion was increased at the next feeding to ensure that when some was left, it signified that the infant had eaten all he or she wanted of it.

The infants were seated in chairs at a low table. All foods were placed in front of the infants on a regular tray without any order in their arrangement. The tray was placed on the low table. Two teaspoons were provided, one for the infant to try to use when it wished, the other for the nurse who sat beside the child. The nurse did not offer food directly or by suggestion. Only when an infant chose a dish, either by reaching or pointing, did a nurse offer a spoonful and only if the infant opened its mouth for that food was the food put in. When the child had definitely finished eating, usually after 20 to 25 minutes, the foods were taken away.

During the course of the experiment, the infants had regular physical examinations, blood tests, urine analysis, and x-ray examinations. They were observed for changes in appetite, evidence of discomfort or abdominal distress after eating, vomiting, constipation, or diarrhea. Stools were examined for undigested food.

The study found that no infant failed to manage their own diet. All of them maintained good appetites. The infants often greeted the arrival of their trays by jumping up and down, and showed impatience while their bibs were being put on. Once placed at the table, having looked the tray over, they usually devoted themselves steadily to eating for 15 or 20 minutes. When their hunger had moderated, they ate intermittently for another five or ten minutes, playing a little with the food, trying to use the spoon, and offering bits to the nurse. None of the infants ever gave any evidence of discomfort or abdominal pain after eating or was constipated. Except in the presence of parenteral infection, there was no vomiting or diarrhea.

There was no clue as to what influenced the infants in choosing the foods they tried and whether the choice was a random one or whether they were attracted by color or odor. It was clear that after the first few meals, the foods most desired were promptly recognized and chosen.

The infants reached without hesitation no matter where the desired food was located on the tray, ignoring other foods that were nearer at hand or brighter in color. Each infant in the beginning chose some foods that he or she spat out after tasting. The infant did not choose these foods again, demonstrating that even by this age, infants develop specific tastes.

Every infant ended up with a unique diet, different from every other infant. None of the diets were predominantly cereal and milk with smaller amounts of fruit, eggs, and meat — which is usually considered optimal meals for this age group. Their tastes changed unpredictably from time to time. Although they showed decided preferences, it proved impossible to predict what any infant would eat at a given meal. Even the daily consumption of milk varied from 11 to 48 ounces. They ate salt only occasionally, often sputtering, choking and/or even crying bitterly after putting it in the mouth but never spitting it out and frequently going back for more, repeating the same reactions.

One of the most striking results was that meals often consisted of strange combinations by adult standards. For example, a breakfast of orange juice and liver, a dinner of eggs and milk. A tendency was seen in all the infants to eat certain foods in waves, i.e., after eating cereals, eggs, meats, or fruits in small or moderate amounts for a number of days, an infant would follow that with a period of a week or longer in which a particular food or class of foods was eaten in larger and larger quantities until astonishingly large amounts were consumed. After this, the quantities would decline to the previous level. The infants did not show any clear preference between raw and cooked foods. Attempts to mix foods or pour milk over any were not observed. Several solid foods were usually taken at each meal, and liquids — milk, orange juice, and water — were drunk at intervals during the course of the meal, as is the habit with adults.

The average daily calories consumed in the diets were found to be within the limits set by scientific nutritional standards for the infant's age and body weight, except in the few instances in which the infants who were undernourished before weaning exceeded the standard when they entered the study.

Five infants had rickets when they entered the study, reflecting a defective deposition of calcium during bone formation. Since vitamin D plays an important role in bone formation, Dr. Davis decided to put cod liver oil, a rich source of vitamin D, on the trays along with other foods. One child with rickets voluntarily drank 178 cc. of pure cod liver oil and 80 cc. of cod liver-incorporated milk in 101 days. About the time the blood calcium and phosphorus reached normal levels and bone x-rays showed the rickets to be healed, he stopped drinking these.

Regardless of their condition at the time of entry to the study, within a reasonable period, the nutrition of all infants improved based on physical examination, urinalysis, blood counts, and bone x-rays. The examining pediatrician commented that they were a fine group of children from both a physical and a behavioral standpoint.

The striking conclusions about the brain's role in our eating habits

While this study was conducted over 70 years ago, the results seem to confirm that humans have a natural regulatory mechanism in the brain that helps us know what we should be eating to obtain our nutritional requirements. For example, the infant's eating a food in increasing volume for a few days and then decreasing the quantity proves the presence of a mechanism that dictates the choice and amount eaten until the immediate nutrient need is met. Taste preferences did not seem as important among the infants as some type of regulatory information telling them what foods their body needed.

Even the body's need for salt became obvious in the experiment. While the infants invariably expressed displeasure at eating raw salt, they consumed it voluntarily, even when another food with less salt and more obvious palatability, Ry-Krisp, was readily available. This suggests the presence of a mechanism to choose food with the maximum concentration of the needed nutrient, salt, from among the items available.

It would also seem that the one infant with rickets who voluntarily partook of cod liver oil validates the presence of a sophisticated regulatory mechanism capable of monitoring nutrient levels inside the body and even identifying nutrients needed to cure a specific defect. After consuming cod liver oil the first time, the infant's choice to keep consuming it seems to show that the brain could identify the food as having the nutrient he needed, then monitor the quantity of the nutrient necessary to consume until his rickets were cured.

ADJUSTING YOUR DIABETIC MEDICATIONS AS YOU IMPLEMENT THE 8 STEPS

PRACTICALLY almost all the glucose in your blood comes from the food you eat, especially grain-based carbohydrates. At present, it is largely the overconsumption of carbohydrates that drives high blood sugar in most countries around the world. However, if no carbohydrate is consumed with a meal, the liver can convert up to 50% of the amino acids absorbed from meat, steak for example, into glucose.

Endocrinologists, by setting the criteria for the diagnosis and management, have made medical treatment of Type 2 diabetes more complicated than it ought to be. For example, if your blood sugar levels keep climbing despite your taking medications, you may be told, without any additional testing, that it is not an indication of your diabetes getting worse. It is because, they tell you, your medications "stopped working" for reasons diabetes experts don't fully understand. If you raise any concern regarding the amount of carbohydrate you are consuming, you may be reassured that carbohydrate is an important nutrient and, as long as the amount per meal/snack does not exceed the recommendation by the experts, you have no reason to reduce it.

They insist that what is needed is to change your medication, use a different combination of medications, start injecting medications that release insulin from your own pancreas, or start you on insulin, along with more frequent tests at home and in the laboratory for monitoring blood sugar levels.

None of those solutions is accurate. If your goal is to lower your blood sugar, reduce or get off your blood sugar medications, and even reverse a diagnosed case of diabetes, you should consider the following steps:

1. *Significantly reduce grain products from your daily diet.* Stop eating bread, pasta, rice, pastries and cakes, and other elements of meals made with starch. *Making lentils the source of carbohydrate for your body is the most effective treatment to reduce elevated blood sugar level if you have prediabetes or diabetes.* Legumes such as lentils were part of the human diet long before agriculture became established as an integral part of human life. The variety of lentils, available in different parts of the world, provides a wider source of needed nutrients compared to the smaller number of cultivated grains.

Remember that, during infancy, most of the excess glucose that was converted to fat in your body came from milk. Your body could make use of the stored fat for your growth, mostly vertical as you grew in height. During adult life, excess glucose, mostly from grains, accumulates in the body as fat and is responsible for your horizontal growth as you gain weight. Since the accumulation of fat leads to the subsequent elevation of blood glucose in a manner that is directly proportional to your intake of carbohydrate, you will see an almost immediate reduction in your blood sugar level, once you significantly reduce grain products from your diet.

2. *Check your fasting blood sugar daily at home until the* levels stabilize within the normal range. (Fasting means not having eaten food for at least ten hours.)

3. *Let your doctor know that you have changed your diet.* Discuss the recommendations in this book with your physician and seek his or her help to lower the dosage of your diabetic medications.

4. *Have your doctor check your fasting blood sugar and triglyceride levels through a blood laboratory.* You may have to pay for this, as your insurance carrier may not approve payment if you are tested more often than they allow. Consult your doctor to decide on the frequency of this test. Your doctor may want to continue testing your A1C levels every three months until he or she is satisfied that you are no longer a diabetic.

How fast your blood sugar will drop is unpredictable because it depends on many factors, including the amount of carbohydrate you are consuming not just in grains, but also in vegetables, fruits, dairy products, and natural sugars.

As you contemplate getting off your medications for diabetes, it is motivating to imagine all the benefits. First, consider the joy of living free of the fear of spending the rest of your life coping with diabetes and its complications. Next, consider the freedom you will experience in not having to carry food with you each time you travel or make sure food is available at your destination, if needed in a hurry. The most common forms of hypoglycemia in Type 2 diabetes occur as a complication of treatments with insulin or other medications. Think how much you will enjoy eating without the restraints imposed by medications, approved foods, or prescribed meal schedules. Also, you will spend less money on medications, blood sugar testing, and doctor visits.

Committing to a new diet will give you the additional benefit of a lower blood triglyceride count with the reduced potential for causing blockage of arteries. In addition, less circulating blood sugar means less water in the circulation to keep the sugar dissolved. This could lead to taking less medication to control blood pressure.

THE REAL ROLE OF EXERCISE IN YOUR HEALTH

LACK OF EXERCISE is blamed as one of the causes for the increasing incidence of diabetes around the world, based on the reasoning that glucose not used to generate muscle energy is contributing to the elevation of blood sugar.

On the surface, you would think this makes sense. When you exercise, your muscles send a message to the brain for additional fuel. The brain, in turn, sends a signal to the liver to release glucose not only to supply fuel to muscles, but also to brain cells.

Many people, especially those young in age, do get benefits such as lower blood sugar using exercise as a tool. However, my opinion is that although it is *possible* to reduce blood sugar through exercise and, in the process, reverse diabetes, it is not *probable* that most people can rely on exercise as their primary method to control blood sugar. Here's why.

First, most people simply do not exercise enough to accomplish the goal of spending enough energy to make a significant difference. Exercising burns very few calories relative to one's daily intake. A woman weighing 140 pounds may expend 270 calories by walking 3.5 miles in one hour, 390 calories by riding a bike for one hour and going a distance of 10 to 12 miles, or 430 calories by running 30 minutes at a speed of 7.5 mph. But if she is doing one of these forms of exercise only two or three times per week, all the while consuming 1800 or 2000 calories per day, she will hardly make a dent in depleting her fat cells. The same goes for men, although the numbers are slightly different.

Add to this the fact that exercise itself usually makes people feel hungrier. You go out for a walk, a bike ride, or to the gym and you then return home and eat even more. Exercise often makes people crave sweets, or think they deserve a reward of an ice cream or chocolate. So if your strenuous exercise regimen is accompanied by increased calorie intake, you might even end up adding more sugar to your bloodstream.

Another problem with exercise is that it does not have the same impact as you age. It is very difficult to keep up the level of activity when you have aging muscles. What used to take 20 minutes to burn 300 calories now takes 40 minutes or even an hour since there is a gradual decrease in the ability to maintain skeletal muscle function and mass.

What is exercise good for

I don't advocate exercise as a tool for diabetes management because I believe exercise is neither necessary nor intended for blood sugar control. If exercise were necessary for blood sugar control, then we would all feel the urge to exercise after a sumptuous meal containing carbohydrates, just as we feel the urge to move when listening to music with a strong beat. Instead, most of us feel lethargic after a heavy meal. Conversely, one might assume that a person who is eating but not exercising should be more likely to develop diabetes compared to one who is younger and able to be more physically active, but not everyone does. For example, the incidence of diabetes is increasing in younger populations compared to senior citizens who typically slow down their physical activities.

Don't get me wrong; exercise will help you lower your blood sugar level because active muscle fibers consume glucose without the presence of insulin (whereas inactive muscle fibers need the presence of insulin to begin allowing the entry of glucose). So it is worthwhile to exercise to warm up your muscles, which triggers them to consume glucose.

However, the primary benefit of exercise is to condition the lungs, heart, and muscles, regardless of your sugar levels. Conditioning develops reserve capacity available for use when you need it or when you become sick. For example, an older person who does not exercise may have the capacity to deliver one liter of oxygen per minute to the tissues and a reserve capacity of three to four liters per minute. An athletically fit old person may have twice that much reserve. When an athletically fit older person develops a condition such as pneumonia, he or she has more available respiratory reserves. The same is true of a conditioned heart in an athletic older individual — it can pump more blood with less effort than an unconditioned person and has the reserves to help that person through a serious illness.

Similar reserves can be expected for the actions of other organs and systems in the body of someone who exercises. For example, conditioning allows your muscles to work longer before your brain senses the stress of exercise and makes you feel tired, compared to the brain that is not conditioned to exercising muscles. The ability of the human body to cope with unexpected events can be improved if the reserve capacities are maintained.

Additional benefits of exercise come from improved blood circulation that helps the brain to think more creatively and the skin to have a better tone. The sustained elevation of body temperature you get from exercise also improves the immune system and defense mechanisms of the body and makes it easier for the transfer of glucose from the blood into active muscle cells. For many people, the addition of exercise in their daily routines also offers the key to greater psychological happiness and wellbeing, even if their blood sugar levels are high.

My newest book, *The Diabetes-Free Cookbook and Exercise Guide,* includes 12 easy-to-do exercises with links to animated videos to show you how to do them. These exercises will help you stay flexible and contribute to building your sense of balance to prevent accidental falls as you age.

FREQUENTLY ASKED QUESTIONS

EVERY PATIENT, medical care provider, Certified Diabetes Educator, dietician, nutritionist, and medical journalist has been led to believe in the existence of insulin resistance as the causative factor of Type 2 diabetes. Each one appears to lack the courage to question the veracity of the concept either because they believe it or because they themselves are not clear about the science behind it.

This author believes that patients asking questions is the only way to motivate the above people to be more cognizant of what is really happening to diabetic patients treated based on this concept. These are questions that I have often been asked by people. I include them here to deepen the explanations already made in the book or to expand on the information you can benefit from.

What is the origin of the insulin resistance theory?

The evolution of insulin resistance to explain Type 2 diabetes is worth knowing because once you see its origin, you can see why it does not appear to be correct.

Originally, it was thought that high blood sugar in adults was similar to that in children, i.e., a lack of insulin production by the pancreas, preventing utilization of glucose by body cells. Thus, it was originally called "adult-onset diabetes." However, when it was found that adults with elevated glucose levels had plenty of insulin, the terminology was changed to "non-insulin-dependent diabetes," as medical science did not understand the reason for the high blood sugar. Eventually, around the 1930s, it was found that some patients, injected with insulin, still had high blood sugar. This led Dr. Wilhem Falta of Vienna to wonder whether body cells are "resistant" to insulin. In the absence of another credible explanation, endocrinologists accepted this hypothesis, commonly known as "insulin resistance."

Oddly enough, medical science has not yet been able to explain why this supposed insulin resistance occurs, nor by exactly what biological mechanism it happens. It remains unexplained why billions of cells suddenly switch to resisting the presence of insulin and prevent glucose from entering them when those cells didn't have the problem before.

One of the most suspicious (and biologically illogical) elements of this theory is that insulin resistance does not occur in all the body's cells. There are 200 types of cells in the body, but the theory states that insulin resistance occurs in only three main groups of cells: 1) muscle cells that have not been warmed up (inactive muscle cells), 2) the liver, and 3) fat cells. No matter how much biological science you know or don't know, it is clear this theory does not make sense. Why would only three types of cells become resistant to insulin?

In addition, there is no finding of any agents that block insulin nor any proof of cellular changes. No research has discovered or demonstrated an actual agent that blocks the binding of insulin with the insulin receptor on cells at the time Type 2 diabetes is diagnosed. In contrast, with many diseases, an agent such as an antibody has been found to block the utilization of molecules in cells. Similarly, there is no proof of any type of change in cells that might make them suddenly resist insulin. Research has not identified any differences in cells that are supposedly insulin resistant and those that are not.

Finally, it is not logical that millions of people around the world are evolving to have resistance to a natural body hormone. The incidence of diabetes is increasing in every nation in the world. It does not make sense that some humans, but not all, in these countries are evolving in a very short time to be resistant to a natural body hormone that helps them utilize glucose as fuel for energy. Diabetes is not a contagious disease, and no other hormones are being affected to the extent we see among the increasing numbers of people developing diabetes.

I suggest you must also consider the illogical paradox of how modern medicine treats Type 2 diabetes in many patients with insulin injections. In no other disease, such as a bacterial infection, do doctors regularly prescribe an antibiotic that the patient is resistant to. For example, have you ever heard of a doctor prescribing even more penicillin to a patient with an infection if the germ is found resistant to penicillin? Yet, endocrinologists have for decades promoted and popularized the idea of using insulin for blood sugar control along with diet and exercise.

A final question to ponder: If insulin injections supposedly help people with Type 2 diabetes with strict control of their blood sugar level, why do so many of them face severe consequences of diabetes? Type 2 diabetics, even those on insulin, have a 50% chance of sustaining damage to kidney function, a 25% chance of complications related to vision, and an increased chance of sustaining complications related to the heart, blood vessels, limbs, and brain functions, compared to people without diabetes. In addition, there is a 25% chance of developing complications associated with low blood sugar caused by insulin injections.

There is no question that sustained blood glucose elevation can lead to a dangerous and even life-threatening condition, because excessive amounts of glucose can cause damage to various types of cells in the body, including nerve cells and cells in the blood vessels, heart, kidney, and eyes. However, the complications sustained by organs following damage to the cells lining the blood vessels come mainly from blockages caused by deposits of fat such as cholesterol and triglyceride. Most people are unaware that when they use insulin to lower their blood sugar level, the glucose removed from the blood is converted to these fat molecules, thus increasing your chances of blood vessel blockages.

This could explain why according to the US National Institute of Diabetes and Digestive and Kidney Diseases, heart disease and stroke are the two leading causes of death among adults with diabetes. This is because narrow blood vessels make it harder for the heart to effectively pump oxygen-rich blood throughout the body. If a blood vessel leading to the brain gets blocked, it can lead to a stroke.

In fact, from 2017 to 2020, there were over one million deaths in the US either directly due to Type 2 diabetes or from its being a contributing cause. Endocrinologists explain away these findings as the manifestations of the progressive nature of Type 2 diabetes, without clarifying why control of blood sugar with insulin injections did not prevent the progression of diabetes.

Why do you say that diabetes is a lifestyle situation?

In my view, Type 2 diabetes is clearly a lifestyle situation, not a hormonal disease. Consider a few examples that go a long way towards proving that lifestyle is at the root of high blood sugar.

When Native Americans were moved to reservations in many states in the 1800s and 1900s, they often received complete physical examinations. The records of these show that from 1832–1939, Type 2 diabetes was extremely rare among Native Americans. However, after living on these reservations, Type 2 diabetes in Native Americans occurred in 16% of the population, compared to a just 8% among

Whites. It was clear that genetic changes did not explain this level of incidence. The most obvious cause was the lifestyle change they underwent, particularly the profound dietary change Native Americans underwent in eating "westernized food," especially the grain-based complex carbohydrates that they were given on the reservations. Compare it to their ancestral way of living, when Native Americans did not cultivate grains but hunted, fished, and farmed crops other than grains like wheat.

The results of a study of dietary changes in 18,090 adults by the Indian Council of Medical Research, published on August 27, 2022, give further evidence. The study had some of the adults eating a control diet consisting of 65–70% carbohydrates and little protein or fat. Meanwhile, the other adults had a diet consisting of 54–57% carbs, 16–20% protein, and 20–24% fat. This simple dietary change of reducing the daily carbohydrate intake by just 8–16%, mostly coming from eating less rice and wheat, resulted in these people significantly lowering their blood sugar levels. This minimal dietary change is what can produce the results you are hoping for.

The current US guidelines for dietary changes for blood sugar control recommend reducing your intake of refined sugar, but this sidesteps the most significant source of blood sugar elevation in the modern-day meal: *complex carbohydrates from grain-based items*. In fact, the dietary guidelines even encourage people to consume whole grains — the very food item that contains more glucose molecules than refined sugar, gram for gram.

What is the connection between Type 2 diabetes, weight gain, and obesity?

In the United States, approximately 85% of people with Type 2 diabetes are overweight or obese. What is the connection? And which comes first — obesity or Type 2 diabetes?

According to the "insulin resistance" theory, it is suggested that the location of fat accumulation in the abdomen predisposes one to develop Type 2 diabetes. But to date, no one has demonstrated a difference in the type of fat stored in the abdominal fat cells vs. other fat cells in the body. Nor has anyone demonstrated that a difference in their metabolic functions among fat cells accounts for the development of Type 2 diabetes. So this simplistic theory of the connection between abdominal fat and diabetes seems unlikely.

I have a different explanation for the association of weight gain and Type 2 diabetes. I suggest that weight gain occurs when adults consume an excess of calories that the body is forced to store as fat, which could be anywhere in the body, not just the abdomen. In the modern diet, the culprit in a high calorie diet is most often complex carbohydrates — grains and grain-flour foods — for some people, 50% or more of their daily caloric intake. When digested, complex carbohydrates release glucose that enters the bloodstream. After cells have absorbed whatever glucose they need under the direction of insulin, the liver keeps a small amount in the form of glycogen, to be released back into the blood if the blood glucose level falls low, such as before lunch or dinner time. But the rest of the excess glucose is converted into fatty acids for long-term storage in our fat cells. If this fat is not burned off through exercise at some later time, it results in gradual weight gain — and eventually obesity.

Meanwhile, it also occurs in many overweight or obese individuals that their fat cell storage eventually fills up. When it happens, the fatty acids remain in circulation in the bloodstream, and as I have suggested, muscle cells begin using those fatty acids for their fuel rather than glucose. This is similar to a car with a hybrid engine using either gasoline or electricity to power the engine. I call this natural change the "fatty acid burn switch." The result: the burning of fatty acids leaves glucose in the bloodstream, leading to high blood sugar (hyperglycemia) and eventually, Type 2 diabetes.

This is the real connection between obesity and Type 2 diabetes. But this is also why even thin people can develop diabetes. Each person has a certain amount of fat storage capacity based on their body type. Thin people can equally fill their smaller fat cells, and while they do not become obese, they may equally develop Type 2 diabetes when their fat storage capacity is filled, leaving glucose in the blood. The same mechanism can also explain gestational diabetes that affects 10% of pregnant women.

Does reducing body weight lead to lower blood sugar?

There is no question that reducing body weight leads to lower blood sugar levels. This is a recognized fact in the traditional treatment of Type 2 diabetes, although endocrinologists cannot explain why. While they claim that being overweight triggers insulin resistance, they are unable to explain the reverse because they will not say that insulin resistance disappears if you lose weight.

As per my theory on the cause of Type 2 diabetes, the connection becomes clear. By losing weight, you empty your fat cells of fatty acids that are being utilized for cellular energy. Eventually, your muscle cells will begin functioning by burning glucose, lowering your blood sugar.

How much weight do you need to lose to begin lowering your blood sugar? I believe that the body has a natural "zone" of balance in which it functions at optimum levels to keep your blood sugar at the right level while providing you with enough energy for your daily functions. I call this zone your "authentic weight." If you are overweight or obese, getting back to your authentic weight and maintaining it requires you to moderate your food intake to the amount of calories that your body can use before the next meal.

How can you know this? In my view, each of us truly has a sense of our authentic weight because our brain tells us what it should be. Let me ask you right now: "What is your authentic weight"? If you focus on answering the question, it is likely that you can get a good sense of what you should weigh. Paying attention to your authentic weight is your brain's way of signaling that you are healthy or that you are exceeding the right weight for you. When you are in tune with your authentic weight, you immediately know it if you gain an extra kilo. You start to feel uncomfortable; you sense your gut is pulling on your muscles. You feel sluggish and tired.

In my view, you cannot rely on standardized tables of height and weight to know your authentic weight. Standardized weight tables are based on average weights of thousands of people and usually have a wide range of pounds in each category. How can you know whether you should be at the lower or the upper end of that range?

Nor can you count on your BMI (body mass index) to determine your weight. In June 2023, the American Medical Association suggested that BMI, commonly used to categorize a person as underweight, normal weight, overweight or obese based on weight and height, does not directly assess the effects of body fat mass on medical conditions such as hypertension and cardiovascular diseases at the individual level. The reason for this is that BMI does not take into account the impact of comorbidities, lifestyle issues, gender, ethnicities, familial conditions, and aging on health. Yet another reason is the influence of eating disorders on fat accumulation. This suggests the need to reevaluate the impact of obesity in other situations such as insulin resistance that leads to high blood sugar, high serum triglycerides and polycystic ovary syndrome (PCOS).

Your authentic body weight is a measure of the total mass of all components of your body, including bone, muscle, organs, blood, fat, and water. The role of each of these components of the body in contributing to one's weight differs in every individual in the world. Two people — one tall and small-boned with lots of muscle and another short and big-boned with regular muscle — could weigh the same. Only you can intuitively know your authentic weight based on what your brain assesses.

Your authentic weight can also change as you exercise and age, because the contributions of each component of weight can change. If you begin working out, adding muscle, you might gain muscle weight but your brain knows you are still in your authentic range because it considers your extra muscle mass. When you age and lose muscle, but gain 10 pounds in body fat, your brain will sense that your authentic weight is now largely composed of fat even though you may weigh the same.

To avoid Type 2 diabetes, your goal must be to take back control of your body and reclaim your authentic weight. If you are unable to rediscover your authentic weight, you can consider the body weight you had when you were in your mid-20s as a close approximation of it, provided your blood sugar and triglyceride levels were within normal range at that time. That is the age at which you might have probably reached your full height and your bones reached their maximum density. Any weight gain after that age reflects in general the increase in pounds you have added due to storing fat and/or building muscle. (For most people, as they age, weight gain is due to storing fat!)

Why do people overeat?

Nearly all weight loss programs are based on the same premise: cut down your intake of food calories and/or increase your exercise in order to burn more calories. Effectively, they all use the same "calories-in calories-out" approach.

This can be effective for some people for some amount of time, but it does not work for everyone. Even for those people who achieve their weight loss goal, it usually does not stick in the long run. They have cravings for foods that they really enjoyed in the past, or they travel and want to try new foods, or they attend parties and family get-togethers, where it is almost impossible to resist eating, regardless of their willpower. Gradually they fall back to their old way of eating and regain the weight they lost, and perhaps gain even more.

I suggest it helps to understand and reflect seriously on why you are tempted to eat more food than your body needs from meal to meal. This means that you have to pay attention to the reason why you decide to eat any meal, however small it may be. Here is a summary of three reasons why people overeat; think about whether you are prone to any of these rather than eating only when your body sends you the hunger signal, which I will discuss in the next FAQ.

1. *Eating for the pure enjoyment of it, even when you are not hungry.*

I suggest that non-hunger eating begins as a temporary and occasional event, done without recognizing its long-range ramifications. It then becomes a habit based on one's enjoyment of food, an experience that triggers the brain to generate dopamine, the pleasure hormone. Here's what happens.

In many adults, the habit of overeating starts as being incidental to other events, such as family picnics or holiday dinners, or any other social occasion with others. It is not a deliberate act of overeating, but a random occurrence. The brain forms a connection between eating and enjoyment. The more these "extra" eating events occur in one's early life, the more the connection is reinforced. Whether you are hungry or not, if food is available and appealing, you learn to feel that it is good to eat it without any consequences.

Little by little, you begin to rationalize overeating in these circumstances. The enjoyment of discovering new foods and the pleasure of eating them, as well as the association of food with positive memories, eventually overcomes your natural inclination to wait to eat until you truly feel hungry. In this way, you begin to establish a behavior of eating when simply stimulated by the sight, smell, or even just the thought of food rather than by your body's hunger signals. The connection between food and enjoyment is stored in your memory and expresses itself without any conscious or deliberate effort. Smelling food being cooked, walking into a colorful supermarket, passing by a restaurant — all these trigger a pleasurable feeling caused by the release of the neurohormone *dopamine*, and you are prompted to want food. You look forward to enjoying a variety of good quality, tasty foods. Or you get a craving for one food in particular.

Once this rationale is established, even your awareness of potential adverse long-term consequences such as weight gain, high blood sugar, high blood cholesterol, or high blood pressure may not be a sufficient deterrent to prevent you from overeating. The behavior continues, even when the consequences are damaging.

2. *Eating when hungry at first, then overeating until your stomach feels full.*

You may start eating in response to the sensation of hunger but rather than stopping when your hunger is satisfied, you don't stop eating until your stomach feels full and almost uncomfortable. You may have started this way accidentally by overeating at family events, parties, business meetings, or trips to new places where food is inexpensive, or you are allowed to eat all you can for the same price. Think about this: most people don't drink until their stomach is full; they stop when their thirst is quenched. But the more times you eat until you feel full, rather than satiated, the more you begin to expect that full feeling. Overeating ensues and it becomes harder to achieve and maintain your authentic weight.

3. *Eating to relieve stress and anxiety.*

Stress is a stimulus that you consider harmful to your safety, security, and wellbeing. People often experience stress as the result of two powerful feelings: fear and pain. This, in turn, induces the stress response that results in the release of hormones such as adrenaline and cortisol. Eating food can lower the amount of adrenaline released, and thus a person who is stressed may turn to food to mitigate the unpleasant effects of stress in the body.

People who tend to overeat often do so for two or three of these reasons rather than just one. The commonality among these is that they all demonstrate that when we overeat, we override the brain's hunger and satisfaction signals.

What are the body's hunger and satiation mechanisms?

To understand hunger, you don't need to look any farther than the mechanism by which babies regulate their consumption of milk, or toddlers regulate their consumption of food. If you think about it, both infants and toddlers decide on their own when to eat, what to eat, and how much to eat to thrive physically, mentally, and emotionally. When you were an infant and then a toddler, this is what you did. So today, to lose weight, you need to alter your eating habits, so you can eat as you did decades ago. I call it "eating like a toddler."

Infants and toddlers only eat in response to the "hunger signal." And they stop eating in response to the "satiation signal." They do not keep eating even if there is food left on the plate. Let me define these two signals.

Hunger signal: Have you ever wondered about the fact that you can never predict precisely when you are going to feel hungry? You probably know, logically and from experience, that you tend to eat every few hours, but what causes the brain to generate the actual sensation of hunger? I suggest that hunger is the feeling that the brain produces to indicate when your body needs nutrients. However, with the body needing over 100 different nutrients for healthy functioning, what makes the brain decide when to create the sensation of hunger?

In my view, it is likely that the brain is responding to cells throughout the body, calling for a variety of nutrients, not just a single one. When the total need of nutrients reaches some threshold level, the brain generates that very recognizable sensation of hunger you feel. To lose weight, see if you can avoid eating until you truly feel hungry.

Satiation signal: As I have already mentioned, we usually do not drink liquids until our stomach is full. We stop drinking when our thirst is quenched, according to a signal the brain sends us. Similarly, the brain actually sends us a signal that we have eaten enough. If you pay attention to chewing your food, you will notice that the taste of the food you are eating becomes less and less enjoyable. This is the brain telling you that, for the present moment, enough needed nutrients from that food have entered the body.

The problem is, most of us get used to eating until our stomach is full. Even if we do not enjoy the food as much as those first bites, we keep eating until the stomach sends a signal to the brain, saying "Enough, I can't take in anymore, please stop." This is effectively a backup signal that the brain sends to stop eating.

Why do so many people disregard the loss of enjoyment signal and keep eating until the full stomach signal alerts them? In my view, it has to do with the habit of overeating we have developed, for any or all of the three reasons cited above, in our youth when there appear to be no consequences. The brain can't alert you during a meal to the long-term consequences of overeating. We do not usually gain much weight at that age, nor incur high blood sugar, so we start believing that overeating is all right once in a while. Later it becomes a regular eating pattern.

To lose weight, you must therefore become conscious of when you are truly hungry and when your brain signals you to stop eating. Think, as I have said, that you need to start "eating like a toddler."

I want to make the transition from grains, but what can I eat?

The ancestors of modern humans appeared on earth about 300,000 years ago. Consumption of wild grains started only after about 200,000 years of human existence and the domestication of rice and grains like wheat and rye dates back to only about 10,000 BCE. This means that humans survived without consuming significant amounts of grain and grain products for the majority of human life on earth.

If you want to eat grains, I suggest that you emphasize alternatives to wheat, rice, and corn. The table here shows how much carbohydrate, fiber, fat, and protein (in grams) is contained in a variety of grains per 100 grams.

Grain	Carbohydrate	Fiber content	Fat content	Protein
White rice	91	1	1	7
Wheat	82	1.2	1.5	12.6
Corn	82	3	1	3
Oats	66	11.6	6.9	16.9
Quinoa	64	7	1.9	14.1
Millet	54	22.6	1.0	7.4

As you can see, if you begin substituting oats, quinoa, and millet in your diet for wheat, rice, and corn, you will obtain the benefits of less carbohydrate, more fiber, more fat, and more protein.

Once you become comfortable with the above, you can attempt further reduction of complex carbohydrates by substituting the following whenever possible.

- *Almond flour* — With a consistency like corn meal, almond flour can be used in pastry, confectionary, and other baking items. Per 100 grams, almond flour contains 21.6 g carbohydrates, 12.5 g dietary fiber, 49.9 g fat, and 21.2 g protein.
- *Chickpea flour* — Also known as besan, this is a pulse flour made from a variety of ground chickpea called Bengal gram or kaalachana. Per 100 grams, it contains 57 g carbohydrates, 10 g dietary fiber, 6 g fat and 22 g protein.

- *Cauliflower flour* — This is an alternative to rice flour. Per 100 grams, it contains 5 g carbohydrates, 2 g dietary fiber, 0.3 g fat and 1.9 g protein.

What other practical suggestions do you have for things I can do to lose weight?

I recommend the following simple changes to your eating habits:

1. As much as possible, during each meal, eat food items that require chewing. Studies suggest that increasing the number of chews per bite increases relevant intestinal signals and may decrease self-reported hunger and food intake. In other words, continued chewing sends more signals from the mouth to the food intake control centers in the brain, facilitating more enjoyment related to that food, and later leading to moderation of the intensity of hunger, thus creating the feeling of satisfaction that allows you to terminate the act of eating and reduce total food energy intake.

2. Sipping warm water every few minutes during a meal cleans the taste buds, creating more contact points for nutrient registration and signal generation to the brain.

3. Concentrate on vegetable preparations that need chewing, rather than blended and pureed foods which do not allow for chewing.

4. To increase chewing, add nuts to certain dishes, or serve on the side.

5. Severely limit the consumption of refined grains and food items made with refined grain-flour that require practically no chewing. From a nutritional point of view, foods made with refined grains and refined grain-flour are empty-calorie foods. If you plan to eat grains or grain-flour-based foods, use whole

grain products instead. To reduce the consumption of glu-
cose-releasing foods, limit the intake of grain-based food items
such as bread, rolls, pasta, cookies, cakes, etc. to not more than
200 of the 570 calories of a single meal.

6. Prepare food items you plan to eat at home, rather than buying
ready-made or pre-packaged. This will give you a head start to
limit your intake of total daily food energy and grain-based
food items. An additional benefit is limiting your intake of
salt.

What causes weight regain after weight loss?

In general, weight reduction programs that include individual or group
counselling to modify how much you eat result in only a 5–10% weight
loss. Unfortunately, as statistics reveal, after six to twelve months following the completion of such a program, most people start regaining
the weight.

Experts suggest many possible reasons for this finding, though
they seldom provide any evidence. For example, one theory states
that weight loss reduces the rate at which your body burns calories.
This then, the theory says, makes it difficult to lose more weight over
a period of months. It seems illogical, though, as it implies that losing
weight has a cap on how much can be lost.

Other theories suggest that a rate of weight loss larger than one or
two pounds per week results in the failure of long-term maintenance
of the reduced weight. For example, most people who lose a large
amount of weight rapidly regain it two to three years later. Why? The
theorists do not explain it.

Let me suggest a few possible logical reasons for regaining lost
weight. First, let's consider motivation. It is normal to be enthusiastic
about any new endeavor, and that enthusiasm makes it easy to commit to a goal. Losing weight as part of an organized program helps

motivate you to accomplish your objective. However, gradually you may find yourself slowly beginning to miss the way you were eating before, or the type and quantity of food you used to eat, so you slide back into your former way of eating, regaining the lost weight. This is demotivating and a real challenge to your sense of commitment.

If you lost weight with the help of medications that modified your natural control mechanisms, terminating the medications could cause a reset of the brain's control mechanisms regarding how hungry you feel and how much you need to eat. This can then result in regaining the lost weight.

The best way to avoid regaining weight is, as explained above, to remain conscious of why you are eating. Are you truly hungry? Or are you eating food out of a need to enjoy it, or out of stress or other emotions, or eating until your stomach feels full rather than being truly satiated?

I also suggest you build the following habits into your daily routine. Check your weight every day around the same time and adjust your food intake for the next 24 hours based on noticing any weight gain. Be aware that you sometimes will have unexpected weight swings due to an excess intake of salt. This causes your body to retain water in order to keep the salt concentration optimal for proper cellular functioning. For this reason, many programs will advise you to weigh yourself no more often than every few days, or only once a week or month. However, it is important to stay consistent in order to see potential issues as soon as possible.

Take pride in yourself when you have a day that shows no weight gain. Notice what you ate the day before that helped you avoid putting on a pound or two. If you put on weight, try eating a large salad for lunch or dinner in place of your usual big meal to lose that extra pound you gained the day before.

Of course, I do agree that it's okay to allow yourself to have an occasional large meal now and again if you have an event or holiday gathering. But if you know you are going to overeat at an event, pre-plan and adjust your food intake during the few days before it. And always be aware of your intake of grains.

What is the connection between a sedentary lifestyle and diabetes?

Experts suggest that sedentary lifestyle and dietary habits are the major factors for the rising incidence of Type 2 diabetes.

A study carried out for a period of six years among more than a thousand nondiabetic individuals from the high-risk population of Pima Indians found that the diabetes incidence rate remained higher in less active men and women from all BMI groups.

Experts suggest that reduced insulin sensitivity in physically less active people leads to the development of diabetes. However, there is no clear explanation of the mechanism by which physical inactivity contributes to the development of Type 2 diabetes.

On the other hand, a CDC report showed that in 2018 there were 28 million people between ages 18–44 diagnosed with prediabetes compared to 24 million people above age 65 in the United States. If physical inactivity was a significant contributor to the development of diabetes, this finding should have been reversed, showing a higher incidence of Type 2 diabetes among the older people. In addition, if it were true that less active people develop insulin insensitivity and diabetes, nearly all elderly people living in retirement facilities should be diabetic or at least prediabetic. But there is no evidence to show this is the case.

In my view, the link between a sedentary lifestyle and diabetes is related to the theory I have proposed as the cause of Type 2 diabetes. As this book suggests, a diet high in grains creates voluminous amounts of glucose in the bloodstream. Any glucose that the body does not utilize immediately (within hours of digesting food) is converted to fatty acids that need to be stored in the fat cells for later use. When the fat cells become full, however, excess fatty acids remain in the bloodstream, to become the primary fuel for muscle cells.

However, if you are sedentary, your muscle cells are not utilizing those fatty acids, neither are they utilizing any glucose created from the foods you digest. The result is the same: excess glucose in the bloodstream, hence high blood sugar (pre-diabetes) and eventually Type 2 diabetes. In both cases, the real cause is a diet that is high in grains and grain-flour products. As to why not all elderly people develop diabetes though they are largely sedentary, the answer is simply that they tend to eat less. It is universally known that the older one gets, the more one's appetite decreases as the body seems to naturally accommodate to less activity.

Why do we need to eat a variety of foods?

Human beings moved from their place of birth to different areas on different continents either to escape inclement living conditions or to reach more favorable living conditions. By surviving in various parts of the earth, humans revealed that there is an abundant availability of nutrients on a timely basis in sufficient quantities for a healthy living. In short, nature has made it possible for humans to survive in almost every part of the globe.

Almost all natural foods from which humans can acquire nutrients come in "containers" made of organic molecules such as cellulose. Think of fruits, vegetables, and nuts. Nature appears to have made these forms of packaging not only to preserve nutrients for the long term, but also to protect food from predators. The packaging in different parts of the globe is different in size, shape, color, aroma, texture, and flavor.

As I pointed out previously in the book, the body needs many nutrients for normal functioning. Science has identified 118 nutrients that are used at some time for human health. No one knows with certainty how much of each of these the body needs or how we derive them from the foods we eat.

That is why I always suggest eating a wide variety of foods to ensure you have the opportunity to ingest as many of these nutrients as possible. It is also why I do not believe in fixed diets or third-party programs that supply you with your meals. Only your brain can tell you what you need to eat at any given meal.

Do artificial sweeteners help control blood sugar?

People with Type 2 diabetes often avoid natural sugar and use artificial sweeteners to lose weight and reduce their blood sugar level. However, this could be counterproductive. Let me explain.

When nutrients such as natural sugar are detected by the receptors in the oral cavity, two alerts are sent: one to the food intake control centers in the brain and the second to the intestine. The brain rewards you by generating the sensation of enjoyment, based on the need for that nutrient in your body at that time. When food reaches the intestine, signals go to the brain, which, in turn, reduces the intensity of enjoyment related to the incoming nutrients to prevent overeating.

Artificial sweeteners, on the other hand, can trigger the sensation of sweet taste. However, they don't appear to be effective in moderating food intake. In fact, evidence shows that long-term use of aspartame, sucralose, stevia, and saccharin leads to weight gain and higher blood sugar levels. This suggests that while the enjoyment of a natural nutrient like sugar is based on the satisfaction of obtain a useful nutrient, the sensation felt with artificial sweetener appears to be based on a conditioned reflex reacting to sweetness from previous experiences. This conditioned response could also explain why some people, addicted to artificial sweeteners, can't enjoy the natural sweetness of fruits without adding artificial sweeteners to them.

Erythritol, a popular artificial sweetener, used in many sugar-free food products, has been linked to increased risk of heart attacks and strokes, according to an article in the February 2023 issue of *Nature Medicine*.[9]

Erythritol is found in very small amounts in fruits and vegetables and is excreted from the body in urine unchanged. People assume that erythritol is safe because it occurs in nature. However, the quantity added to a prepared food can be 1,000 times greater than that seen in natural foods.

The fact is, the natural sugar consumed on average in everyday drinks and foods is not a significant contributor to blood sugar, unless you drink a large amount of soft drinks sweetened with sugar. The main cause of blood sugar elevation in Type 2 diabetes is glucose released after the digestion of complex carbohydrates in grains such as wheat, rice, and corn. Therefore, if you can cut the amount of grain-based foods to one-half of what you are consuming on a daily basis, you can lower your blood sugar and continue to enjoy natural table sugar in your tea, coffee, and your food preparations.

Is natural sugar bad for diabetics?

Many people are confused about whether natural sugar, i.e., sucrose, is the same as glucose in your bloodstream. Sucrose is found in fruits, berries, sugar cane, sugar beets, and other crops that can be boiled down into forms of sugar. The confusion is understandable because, when discussing diabetes, we always refer to the problem of having high blood "sugar." The same word "sugar" appears to be referring to the same item, so there is a tendency among many people to think that eating any natural sugar increases their blood sugar.

For example, many people make pastries with reduced amounts of sugar (sucrose), believing that they can now consume more of the pastries, without realizing that the pastries are likely to put more sugar (glucose) in the blood from the flour used than the sugar they put in their coffee.

Digesting natural sugar (sucrose) is not the same as filling your bloodstream with glucose. Sucrose contains equal parts of glucose and fructose. Both are absorbed as they're released in the intestine. But while the glucose adds to your blood sugar level almost immediately, fructose is absorbed only half as fast as glucose and has to be further processed into glucose before it can elevate your blood sugar level. This means eating a piece of fruit for breakfast or dessert doesn't cause the same level of blood sugar peak, compared to an equal amount of carbohydrate in a grain-based product such as toast, muffins, cake, or pie, so it is effectively healthier for you.

The same is true for milk sugar (lactose), which is made of one molecule of galactose and one molecule of glucose. Galactose must be further processed by the liver before it can elevate your blood sugar. The medical profession has done a poor job of educating people that natural sugar has not been shown to increase the incidence of complications in Type 2 diabetes. In fact, the medical profession might have unwittingly contributed to creating a prevailing culture in which people fear the natural sugars of whole fruit.

Should I eat according to the 2023 Food Pyramid?

The first Food Pyramid was created in the 1970s in Sweden by a special committee to suggest nutritionally balanced meals at a reasonable cost. In 1992, the United States Department of Agriculture (USDA) introduced a Food Pyramid to recommend servings of each food group, which previous guides did not do.

The 2023 Food Pyramid modified the recommendations in an attempt to improve the health of Americans who continued to experience increasing incidence of cardiovascular diseases and Type 2 diabetes. For example, meats are to be consumed monthly or in small amounts compared to the previous recommendation of 2 to 3 servings per day. Eggs, poultry, and dairy are to be taken daily to weekly, compared to prior recommendation of 2 to 3 servings a day. Fish and seafood are to be eaten a few times per week compared to 2 to 3 times per day. Olive oil can be consumed in variable amounts daily compared to sparingly. Fruits and vegetables can be consumed daily compared to 3 to 5 servings per day. Whole grains, bread, legumes, and nuts can be taken daily compared to 6 to 11 servings per day of bread, cereal, rice, and pasta.

In essence, the new Food Pyramid is primarily based on the Mediterranean diet. Overall, that diet is mostly plant-based and focuses on healthy fats that include virgin olive oil, avocados, nuts, salmon, and sardines. Red meat consumption is limited to a few times a month.

As you can see, the emphasis of both the Pyramids, the original and the new USDA version, is on minimizing the intake of dietary fat, especially saturated fat such as cholesterol, which literally creates the plaque that blocks blood passages and leads to heart attacks and strokes.

However, in my opinion the new Pyramid will not help achieve the objective of reducing the incidence of cardiovascular events or Type 2 diabetes. This is because it fails to address the root cause of excess food consumption. For example, the investigators failed to take into consideration that vegetarians who do not consume animal products also get the same cardiovascular diseases. Even more importantly, although the calculation of average intake of food groups can be useful for comparison of study results, it cannot be directly applicable to all individuals because each person's nutrient needs are different.

This major deficiency is what I am trying to offset in this book in order to reverse and prevent Type 2 diabetes through my recommendations. Exercise, weight control, and reducing the consumption of grains and grain-flour products are the keys to avoiding Type 2 diabetes and its myriad complications.

Can meal timing help weight control?

An estimated 33% of the global adult population is classified as overweight. Some researchers looking to lower this number think that "meal timing" can be a viable solution to helping people lose weight.

In some short-duration studies (5–6 weeks only), it has been shown that participants with a high degree of compliance were able to control their weight by consuming more calories in the morning than during the later part of the day. The research suggests that our bodies are primed to metabolize food after the overnight fasting period, and therefore we should eat the majority of our calories during the morning or afternoon. The recommendations also emphasize not to skip breakfast as it could lead to more intense hunger and binge eating later in the day.

Another suggestion is to eat a small dinner early in the evening or at least two to three hours before going to bed. In general, researchers recommend eating this way at least five times a week if it is not possible to do it daily. Researchers claim that these recommendations are based on the natural biological clock in the body that activates physiological mechanisms, including those related to hunger and food intake.

However, I suggest that one does not need to gorge oneself at breakfast. It is understandable that the body activates the hunger mechanism after sleeping due to a need to replenish nutrients. But it is also obvious that the body is not expecting a sudden influx of nutrients. Otherwise, one would feel the greatest intensity of hunger in the morning, which for most people, is not so. The fact that the hunger sensation can be felt at any time of the day means that the body can handle eating for nutrition whenever it is ready for it, regardless of time of the day.

An extreme example of meal timing is intermittent fasting to reduce food calorie intake by eating only on alternate days, not eating on certain days of the week, or restricting eating to specified times of the day. The US National Institute on Aging states that there is insufficient evidence to recommend intermittent fasting for general use although considered harmless. A study published in the *Journal of the American Heart Association* in 2023 concluded that the use of time-determined eating was not helpful as a strategy for long-term weight loss in a general medical population.[10]

Can I have a surgical procedure to lose weight?

In extreme cases, medical practitioners may suggest bariatric surgery, pointing out that most people maintain reduced weight after the surgery. But most such surgical procedures achieve long-term weight loss through one of three mechanisms: decreasing nutrient absorption, restricting food intake, or affecting the body's cell signaling pathways. Often, the procedures affect several of these mechanisms. Let me explain them.

Some procedures reduce the ability of the intestines to absorb nutrients. Though this may help a person lose weight, it can result in deficiencies of iron, vitamin B12, fat soluble vitamins, thiamine, and folate. Inappropriate insulin secretion is another complication of this type of surgery. Yet another complication is deep vein thrombosis with a potential for pulmonary embolism. In addition, rapid weight loss after obesity surgery can contribute to the development of gallstones. Increased incidence of alcohol and mental health related issues have been reported after obesity surgery.

Other procedures restrict your food intake by making the stomach smaller. The gastric bypass, one of the common bariatric surgeries, reduces the size of the stomach by well over 90%, i.e., to about 15 milliliters (ml) in size compared to a normal stomach that can stretch, sometimes to over 1000 ml. What you may not realize is that this procedure helps you lose weight simply because you cannot eat as much as before. So before agreeing to this type of surgery, I suggest you find out how much food someone who had this type of surgery can consume. Then consume a similar amount of food for a while. See if you can achieve similar weight loss and weight maintenance without having to suffer the surgery or its consequences.

Another procedure is thought to effect weight loss by altering the physiology of weight regulation and eating behavior. For example, after surgery, patients are asked to have 5-6 small meals daily, and *not* graze between meals. Meals after surgery are restricted to only ½ - $\frac{1}{4}$, slowly increased to 1 cup over a span of one year.

A warning, as well: After bariatric surgery, people may tend to feel good about themselves for the weight loss, but a significant minority experience psychological complications, including but not limited to grieving the loss of food, regrets about having had surgery, relationship changes, and fear of weight regain. One study that followed up for nearly 40 years on almost 22,000 surgical patients representing the major types of bariatric surgeries showed a reduction in mortality rates, including cardiovascular-, cancer-, and diabetes-related death rates compared to matching controls. However, patients in that study between ages 18–34 had increased mortality following bariatric surgery in relation to suicide, accidents, and cirrhosis of the liver. The authors of the study recommended more research in these areas.

Why can't I take insulin or other drugs to control my blood sugar?

You can use insulin to control your blood sugar and may believe that it will help you escape the usual complications of Type 2 diabetes in the long term. But what may be surprising for most Type 2 diabetic patients is the fact that even if you keep your blood sugar below 7 as indicated by your A1C, you are still likely to develop kidney function failure and increased chances of developing heart, brain, vision, and leg problems, compared to controlling your blood sugar with dietary changes.

Other drugs currently used to control blood sugar work by prolonging the action of the intestinal signaling mechanisms that control your desire for food intake. For example, the intestine releases a hormone in response to glucose molecules in food as soon as you start eating. This hormone then stimulates the pancreas to release insulin to help digest glucose. The hormone also promotes brain action to suppress the sensation of hunger, which is usually degraded within minutes. Pharmaceutical researchers have, therefore, found a way to prolong the action of this intestinal hormone so that it continues to stimulate insulin release and cause a longer suppression of hunger. However, these drugs often cause nausea, vomiting, diarrhea, and constipation in a significant number of people. It is understandable that people with an upset stomach consume less food and lose weight.

Meanwhile, the use of weight loss drugs to control appetite also carries many side effects, one of which is interference with the absorption of necessary nutrients in a timely fashion, which can lead to food cravings.

Will changing my diet increase my lifespan?

It is well recognized that Type 2 diabetes is associated with an overall shorter lifespan. For example, just by reducing A1C (hemoglobin blood sugar) from 9.9% to 7.7%, it has been shown that you might gain 3.4 years in life expectancy.

The concern is that as the age of people diagnosed with Type 2 diabetes goes down (now even occurring in teens and pre-teens), we can expect a further decrease in the lifespan. Unfortunately, diabetologists have no specific strategies to address the increasing incidence of diabetes occurring at younger and younger ages. This is a true tragedy.

As discussed earlier, the metabolic activities inside each cell in the body produce agents known as "Reactive Oxygen Species" (ROS). These agents can cause damage to proteins and/or the genes inside the cell. This is what causes an age-related limit on lifespan due to cellular damage.

There are four possible outcomes when cells sustain gene damage:

1. *Repair and maintenance:* Cells can actually repair genes damaged in their structure and functionality. The greater one's body is able to repair gene damage, the longer one's life span. It has been shown that centenarians 100–107 years old have greater levels of gene repair mechanisms compared to 69–75-year-old individuals in the general population.

2. *Defective functionality:* Without gene repair, the accumulation of damage to genes as humans age not only limits the functional capability of cells, which causes a reduced lifespan, but also leads to a gradual reduction in the quality of life. This occurs because gene damage can limit muscle strength and stamina. One highly visible example of the result of such injury is hair loss as one ages due to gene damage sustained by stem cells in charge of hair renewal.

3. *Uncontrolled activity:* The accumulation of gene damage can also result in uncontrolled cell multiplication, which initiates the formation of a cancer. However, this usually occurs over an extended amount of time, literally decades. The average age of an adult cancer patient is over sixty years. (Note that gene damage resulting in cancer can also be due to factors other than ROS. For example, radiation, exposure to cancer-causing chemicals in cigarettes and in the environment, infections, and chronic inflammation can all lead to either damage to existing genes or mistakes during gene construction.)

4. *Cellular senescence:* When cells have accomplished their assigned tasks, they enter into a state of inactivity called "cellular senescence" (old age), after which cells in the immune system clear them away. However, when the rate of generation of senescent cells exceeds the capability of the immune system to remove them, perhaps due to an age-related decline in immune function, senescent cells can persist. Although they may not be able to perform useful functions, they may remain metabolically active, producing molecules that promote inflammation. For example, scientists link an accumulation of senescent cells in lungs that were exposed to cigarette smoke as contributing to airway inflammation. Exercise has been shown to improve the efficiency of the immune system to remove senescent cells and improve muscle strength in older adults.

In summary, most age-related disabilities stem from the imbalance between cellular damage due to normal metabolic activities and the ability of the immune system to recognize and repair them. One solution is to reduce cellular metabolism, which will limit the production of ROS. The best example of how effective this can be is the lifespan of Greenland sharks, which — barring injury, poison, disease, lack of available resources, changes to environment, or capture — can live between 250 and 500 years. These sharks have the lowest swim speed and tail-beat frequency relative to their size among all fish species, which most likely correlates with their very slow metabolism and extreme longevity.

However, we humans, because of our greater brain capabilities and continuous inputs from our senses, are compelled to engage in activities that create a large amount of ROS.

Nevertheless, there are some mitigating actions that you can take to lower the production of ROS. One significant step is to reduce stress, which helps reduce the production of ROS. With training and practice, you can learn to deal with a stressful event with minimal release of stress hormones. In addition, exercise can help you expend some of the stress hormones released, reducing their impact on metabolic activities that could lead to more ROS generation. Read about stress in the answer to the following question.

What is the role of stress in diabetes?

The word stress generally refers to a force or influence; as applied to the lives of humans, stress refers to any stimulus that alters the meaning or intensity of one's feelings, actions, or communications. Signals that you interpret as harmful to your safety, security, or wellbeing are the ones that cause a stress response. The stimuli that cause stress are essentially the same for most people — perceived threats, illness, injury, overwork, unsolved work issues, family problems, relationship issues, or other inconveniences. The intensity and duration of the stimuli needed to elicit the stress response varies for each person. One individual may be able to handle many difficult life events that another would find highly stressful. The difference appears to be due to the conditioning and training one receives from parents to cope with stress starting in early childhood and continuing to adulthood, which determines a person's sensitivity to stressful stimuli as an adult.

In general, people experience stress as an outcome of two powerful feelings: fear and pain. Fear can be imagined or real and based on known or unforeseen factors. Fear, by definition, is more emotional than rational. During the fear response, neurons located in the primitive core part of the brain (the limbic system) are activated before the stimulus can be analyzed on the intellectual level (in the prefrontal cortex) to determine if it is real and deserves a thoughtful reaction. This fear forces you to determine what to do based on an incomplete analysis of partial information. Pain can be physical or emotional. It can be based on a current event or a past experience.

The time of onset, degree, and duration of the stress response varies with each individual, as determined by the hormones released in the body during the stress response. For instance, let's look at anger, a feeling of displeasure aroused by real or imagined stress. If your body releases adrenaline at the slightest provocation, you're a person who will get angry quickly and easily. If the amount of adrenaline released is large or if your sensitivity to it is high, the intensity of your anger will also be high. If you remain in the stressful environment or dwell on the stress in your mind, your body can continue releasing the hormone for a long period, setting the stage for prolonged anger. If you routinely expect a person or event to create displeasure for you, it may cause you to be angry each time you encounter that person or event.

The role of stress in diabetes is related to two consequences. First, when you are under stress you may react by eating, since the hormone, dopamine, released by the pleasures of eating can counterbalance the stress hormones and lessen the sensation of stress.

Secondly, just receiving a diagnosis of Type 2 diabetes can trigger a continuous sense of stress in many people. In my opinion, the quality of life deteriorates from the moment Type 2 diabetes is diagnosed. The patient is confused about the reason for getting diabetes. Doctors usually ask about the patient's family history of diabetes, and the latter is more likely than not to conclude that it is hereditary because someone in the family has it now or had it. The patient will be asked to lose weight and given instructions not to skip meals while on diabetic medications lest she may suffer symptoms of low blood sugar.

This life change is often stressful for a person who has never experienced symptoms of low blood sugar and therefore is unfamiliar with what they are supposed to feel. A low-level sense of trepidation and fear may become common in the person's life. They may not know what to do when they feel a sharp hunger sensation as a consequence of taking the diabetic medication. Meanwhile, to prevent the consequences of low blood sugar, the doctor may have advised the patient to carry food at all times, especially when access to sugar-containing food is not assured, such as when traveling. Family members and friends may worry about not being able to serve what the person is allowed to eat, or worse, not knowing how to deal with a low blood sugar situation if it occurs. Gradually, the person who has been diagnosed with Type 2 diabetes may decline to go out very much for fear of inconveniencing their friends and family. This could lead to emotional distress and its related stress responses, thus creating further doubts about being able to control one's diabetes.

How does exercise improve the quality of my life?

Remaining physically active as we grow old is the best way to prevent or keep in check lifestyle-related illnesses like diabetes in order to maintain the quality of life and increase our lifespan. A key indicator of the state of one's physical health is the efficiency of the metabolic activities inside each cell. Aging naturally affects that efficiency, by reducing the power generation of mitochondria, which leads to more ROS production. This, in turn, not only increases the chance of lifestyle-associated diseases but also accelerates the aging process. This is precisely why exercise is critical to your quality of life. It has been shown that lifelong exercise training improves mitochondrial efficiency, lowers ROS production, and contributes to healthy aging.

There are many additional health benefits from regular exercise that affect the quality of life. For example, chances are you have never thought about how blood returns to the heart from different parts of the body, even against gravity, for example, from the legs, compared to the heart sending it there by the force of the heartbeat. You may not realize that the return of blood is aided by contractions of muscles that act as pumps to push the blood through the veins. To prevent blood from dropping back under the pull of gravity, veins have valves spaced at different intervals. It is when these valves fail that you see the bulging which creates varicose veins. In addition, if you remain immobile for extended periods of time, such as during air travel or if you are bedridden, blood can stay stagnant, leading to the formation of blood clots that can be dangerous.

To help you with your decision to exercise regularly, let me give you a few suggestions:

1. Be clear about why you want to exercise and what your exact objective is. For example, you might want to feel good about yourself being able to continue and enjoy certain physical activities as long as you can. Or you may want to improve your stamina or build muscle in order to keep up with your grandchildren. Perhaps you simply want to be able to carry out your everyday tasks, such as getting in and out of a car, more easily.

2. Be adaptive. Sometimes you may find it hard to exercise because of travel, illness, or a pressing need for your time; rather than letting this situation discourage you, be adaptive and look forward to the next chance.

3. Connect exercise with something you routinely do. For example, consider exercising every morning after your personal hygiene needs are met or before you settle down in the evening in front of the television.

4. As often as possible, appreciate your ability to continue physical exercise. Patting yourself on the back is both a good literal and motivational exercise.

5. To make physical exercise a part of your daily routine, start slowly, especially if you have been relatively sedentary for a

long time. Create a mindset of curiosity to understand what the exercise you plan to do is and how it can help you. As you gradually master each exercise routine, you will find it increasingly comfortable to do. You will notice positive impacts in all aspects of your life. With commitment and perseverance, you will begin looking forward to exercising with the result that you are missing it when you can't do it on account of travel or other pressing needs.

END NOTES

1. *Are Baby Boomers Healthier than Generation X? A Profile of Australia's Working Generations Using National Health Survey Data.* Pilkington et al. PLoS One 9(3): March 2014

2. Obesity and overweight: World Health Organization https://www.who.int/news-room/fact-sheets/detail/obesity-and-overweight

3. Kannel, WB. 1985. Lipids, diabetes, and coronary heart disease: Insights from the Framingham Study. *American Heart Journal* 110:1100-1107

4. Statin use and risk of diabetes mellitus in postmenopausal women in the *Women's Health Initiative.* Arch Intern Med 2012 Jan 23;172(2):144-52

5. Insulin's ability to lengthen the life span and improve the quality of life of patients with diabetes is clearly established. However, this conclusion is primarily based on the results of treating patients with Type 1 diabetes who suffer progressive damage to insulin-producing cells in the pancreas. The conclusion is less applicable to those taking insulin for Type 2 diabetes.

6. See http://www.nhlbi.nih.gov/guidelines/obesity/BMI/bmicalc.htm.

7. Swithers, SE. 2013, Artificial sweeteners produce the counterintuitive effect of inducing metabolic derangements. *Trends in Endocrinology and Metabolism.* 24:431-441

8. Davis, CM. 1928, Self-selection of diet by newly weaned infants. An experimental study. *The American Journal of Diseases of Children.* 36:651-679.

9. *The artificial sweetener erythritol and cardiovascular event risk.* M. Witkowski, I. Nemet, H. Alamri, et al: Nature Medicine: Feb 2023

10. https://www.ahajournals.org/doi/10.1161/JAHA.122.026484

ABOUT THE AUTHOR

JOHN M. POOTHULLIL, MD, FRCP practiced medicine as a pediatrician and allergist for more than 30 years, with 27 of those years in the state of Texas. He received his medical degree from the University of Kerala, India in 1968, after which he did two years of medical residency in Washington, DC and Phoenix, Arizona, and two years of fellowship, one in Milwaukee, Wisconsin and the other in Ontario, Canada. He began his practice in 1974 and retired in 2008. He holds certifications from the American Board of Pediatrics, The American Board of Allergy & Immunology, and the Canadian Board of Pediatrics. During his medical practice, Dr. Poothullil became interested in understanding the causes of and interconnections between hunger, satiation, and weight gain. His interest turned into a passion and a multi-decade personal study and research project that led him to read many medical journal articles, medical textbooks, and other scholarly works in biology, biochemistry, physiology, endocrinology, and cellular metabolic functions. This eventually guided Dr. Poothullil to investigate the theory of insulin resistance as it relates to diabetes. Recognizing that this theory was illogical, he spent several years rethinking the biology behind high blood sugar and developed the fatty acid burn theory as the real cause of diabetes.

Dr. Poothullil has written articles on hunger and satiation, weight loss, diabetes, and the senses of taste and smell. His articles have been published in medical journals such as *Physiology and Behavior, Neuroscience and Biobehavioral Reviews, Journal of Women's Health, Journal of Applied Research, Nutrition,* and *Nutritional Neuroscience.* His work has been quoted in *Woman's Day, Fitness, Red Book,* and *Woman's World.*

Dr. Poothullil is the author of six books, including this one. Three other books focus on Type 2 diabetes, and are profiled on the following pages. In addition, he has published two books about cancer:

- *Surviving Cancer: A New Perspective on Why Cancer Happens & Your Key Strategies for a Healthy Life* (New Insights Press, 2017)
- *When Your Child Has Cancer: Insights and Information to Empower Parents* (New Insights Press, 2020)

———

Please visit the website DrJohnOnHealth.com to follow
Dr. Poothullil's blog and to send us your questions
and feedback on how this book has changed your life.

OTHER BOOKS ON DIABETES
BY DR. JOHN POOTHULLIL

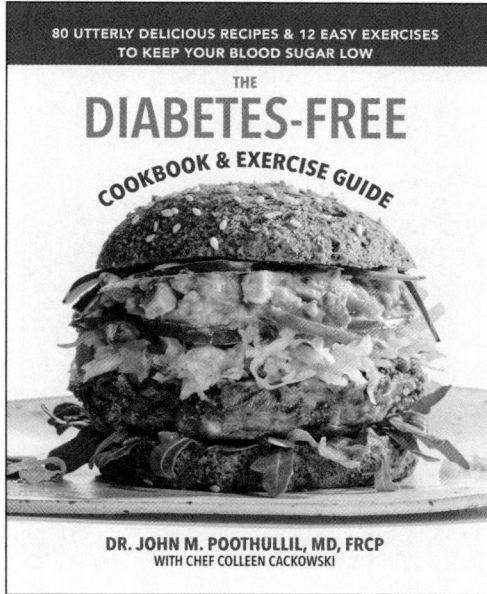

The Diabetes-Free Cookbook and Exercise Guide

Discover how you can live a diabetes-free life with Dr. John's groundbreaking cookbook and exercise guide. With over 80 appetizing low-carb recipes created by Chef Colleen Cackowski, you'll never miss the high-carb, high-sugar foods of your past. Every recipe nourishes your body and keeps your blood sugar levels in check so you can enjoy tasty, satisfying meals. Dr. John also offers 12 easy-to-do exercises to boost your flexibility and balance and keep you healthy as you age.

New Insights Press
Copyright © 2023
ISBN: 979-8-9860163-4-4 (Paperback)
ISBN: 979-8-9860163-7-5 (eBook)

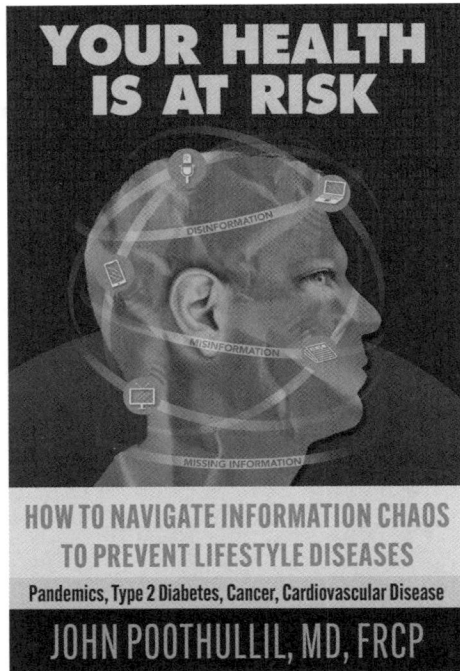

Your Health Is at Risk: How to Navigate Information Chaos to Prevent Lifestyle Diseases

This book explains how medical disinformation, misinformation, and missing Information (DMMI) are increasingly pervasive in the media and social media, leading you to make poor or wrong decisions about your lifestyle choices and healthcare. The book offers insights into how you can make wiser decisions based on science to improve your health.

Gold Medal Winner, 2023 Nautilus Book Awards and Independent Press (Ippy) Awards

New Insights Press
Copyright © 2022
ISBN: 978-1-7359344-7-1

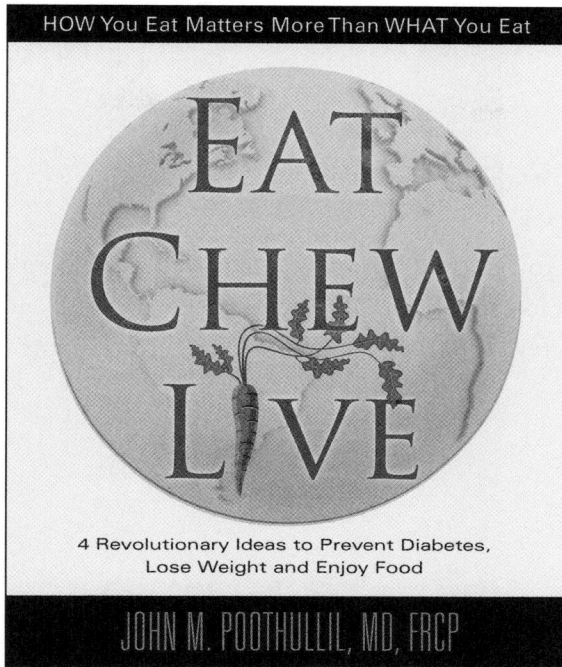

Eat Chew Live: 4 Revolutionary Ideas to Prevent Diabetes, Lose Weight and Enjoy Food

This book goes into extensive detail about the lack of logic with the insulin resistance theory as the cause of high blood sugar and Type 2 diabetes, and what everyone can do to change their thinking and eating habits.

Winner, 2016 Beverly Hills Books Awards

Over and Above Press
Copyright © 2015
ISBN: 978-0-9907924-1-3

If you enjoyed this book or received value from it,
then I'd like to ask you a favor: would you be kind enough to
leave a review of it on Amazon? It'd be greatly appreciated!